Integrity of Randomized Clinical Trials

Today, scientists are expected to be more accountable and transparent than at any other time in history. Globally, the pursuit of knowledge creation enjoys a place of distinction, and the public expects to reap considerable benefits from the innovative contributions made by researchers. It is, therefore, more important than ever that ethics, transparency, and professionalism explicitly guide research integrity.

Despite the clear importance of acquiring a fundamental understanding of clinical trials in the context of health research and innovation, medical training generally fails to cover clinical trial integrity in its curriculum, including it neither at the undergraduate nor at the postgraduate levels. This new book provides a curriculum to address this gap, offering best practice guidelines to improve the quality, openness, and trustworthiness of clinical trials and filling a current void in the market.

Key Features:

- The first book on clinical trial integrity
- Provides clear guidance on how to ensure probity in peer review, appraisal of trials, and investigation of complaints concerning misconduct in clinical trials
- Trains and supports researchers globally on how to undertake trials with integrity
- Ensures that the increasing demand for public documentation of all aspects throughout the lifecycle of a clinical trial can be met

This book is essential reading for master and doctoral students undertaking courses in clinical trials, epidemiology, and medical statistics and an invaluable reference for medical journal editors and peer reviewers, clinicians who recruit patients into trials, pharmaceutical industry profession-als, patient and public representatives who engage in clinical trials, systematic reviewers, guideline writers, and funders and regulators of clinical trials.

Integrity of Randomized Clinical Trials

HOW TO PREVENT RESEARCH MISCONDUCT AND ENSURE TRANSPARENCY

Khalid S. Khan
Beatriz Galindo Distinguished Investigator
University of Granada
Spain

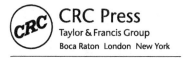

CRC Press
Taylor & Francis Group
Boca Raton London New York

CRC Press is an imprint of the
Taylor & Francis Group, an **informa** business

Designed cover image: gettyimages Credit - Andrew Brookes

First edition published 2025
by CRC Press
2385 NW Executive Center Drive, Suite 320, Boca Raton FL 33431

and by CRC Press
4 Park Square, Milton Park, Abingdon, Oxon, OX14 4RN

CRC Press is an imprint of Taylor & Francis Group, LLC

ISBN: 978-1-032-60986-7 (hbk)
ISBN: 978-1-032-60122-9 (pbk)
ISBN: 978-1-003-46140-1 (ebk)

DOI: 10.1201/9781003461401

Typeset in Rotis
by Deanta Global Publishing Services, Chennai, India

Contents

Preface   vii

About the author   ix

Acknowledgments   xi

Abbreviations   xiii

1   Introduction   1

2   Randomized clinical trials   9

3   Integrity of trials   27

4   Ethics committee approval and participant consent   43

5   Trial planning   62

6   Trial oversight   78

7   Publishing trials responsibly   92

8   Authorship of trials   112

9   Evidence syntheses of randomized clinical trials   126

10 Investigating research misconduct allegations   142

Suggested reading   161

Glossary   162

Index   194

Preface

In July 2023, the *Nature* journal announced that "Medicine is plagued by untrustworthy clinical trials". It challenged the foundational basis of the research evidence behind the interventions used every day in healthcare worldwide. It pointed towards a systems failure.

Clinical trials underpin modern healthcare. They bring about breakthroughs in disease prevention and cure. Around 25,000–30,000 randomized clinical trials are published annually. Evidence-based medicine, the healthcare paradigm that deploys research to inform decision-making and policies, recognizes randomized clinical trials as the most valid form of evidence. However, the number of published trial retractions from the scientific literature is on the rise. Flaws in published trial integrity have downstream consequences. They entail risks to patients and public health. There is public concern about the fundamentals of healthcare research. This issue ought to be addressed at the root cause level.

Where does one start? There are many international research integrity statements, which appear to do little more than pay lip service. From inception to publication, a trial has a long journey passing through the hands of many stakeholders. To name a few steps along the way, trials pass through the hands of human research ethics committees, funding bodies, institutional research governance, independent trial oversight committees, and journal editorial and peer review assessments. All have opportunities to pick up integrity flaws. Retraction of a published randomized clinical trial signals the failure of all of the custodian stakeholders; each must do its own soul-searching. Academic institutions might ask: What went wrong with their research governance? How have they come to fail in the most basic of their duties to supervise the trials conducted under their flag? Journals might ask: Why did their editorial and peer review assessments fail?

Slogans of zero tolerance against scientific fraud are just empty gestures. Business as usual cannot continue. The stakeholder organizations must be prepared to make some substantive changes based on the lessons learned. To address the above challenges, this book will offer best practice guidance to improve the trustworthiness of randomized clinical trials.

Khalid S. Khan

About the author

Khalid S. Khan is Professor of Public Health and Preventive Medicine at the University of Granada, Spain. He is a Distinguished Investigator of the prestigious Beatriz Galindo program of the Spanish Ministry of Education. He has been a Professor at the University of Birmingham and the Queen Mary University of London, UK, and a Spinoza Professor at the University of Amsterdam, the Netherlands. His research expertise has been recognized with his appointment as a Senior Investigator at the UK National Institute of Health Research. He was the founding Director of the World Health Organization Collaborating Centers for Research in Birmingham and London, UK. He has won several prestigious awards, including the Sims Black Fellowship from the Royal College of Obstetricians and Gynecologists, and the Strutt and Harper Grant from the British Medical Association, UK.

Khalid has covered the complete range of trial-related work in his research career spanning three decades. Question formulation, prioritization and protocol development, funding and approvals, trial conduct and data analysis, research governance and audit, independent trial oversight and monitoring, peer review and publication, evidence syntheses and guidelines, consensus development for trial integrity, etc. have all been part of his experience. He has supervised doctoral students working on trials and has examined doctoral theses based on randomized clinical trials in Denmark, Holland, Spain, and the UK. Three of his trainees have directed clinical trial units. He has been a member of grant-giving panels for assessing and awarding trials in the UK and Germany. He has led or co-led as a principal investigator two dozen published trials with over 13 thousand randomized participants. In his role as director of research and development, he has been responsible for the research governance framework. He has undertaken investigations of allegations of scientific misconduct among trials in progress and post-publication. As a journal editor, he has presided over 10 thousand manuscript evaluations. As a scientific author, he has over 500 publications in peer-reviewed research journals. With an *h*-index >100 his work has attracted a high level of citation. He has been ranked consistently amongst the top 2% of the world's most influential scientists.

Acknowledgments

No trialist can develop without the guidance of many. I am most grateful to the late Professor Richard Gray, founding director of the Birmingham Clinical Trials Unit, UK, for mentoring me. This book is dedicated to him. I am grateful to Professor Aurora Bueno-Cavanillas, Department of Public Health and Preventive Medicine, University of Granada, Spain, and Professor Javier Zamora, Clinical Biostatistics Unit, Ramón y Cajal Hospital, Madrid, Spain, for their critical appraisals of the initial drafts of the chapters in this book.

Khalid S. Khan

Abbreviations

ACTIVE	Authors and Consumers Together Impacting on eVidencE
AI	Artificial Intelligence
AMSTAR	A MeaSurement Tool to Assess systematic Reviews
CoARA	Coalition for Advancing Research Assessment
CER	Control Event Rate
CONSORT	CONsolidated Standards Of Reporting Trials
COPE	Committee on Publication Ethics
COVID-19	Coronavirus disease 2019
CRediT	Contributor Roles Taxonomy
DELTA	Difference ELicitation in TriAls
DOAJ	Directory of Open Access Journals
DOI	Digital Object Identifier
DORA	Declaration on Research Assessment
EBM	Evidence-based Medicine
EMA	European Medicines Agency
EQUATOR	Enhancing the QUAlity and Transparency Of health Research
FAIR	Findable, Accessible, Interoperable, and Reusable data sharing
FDA	The US Food and Drug Administration
GCP	Good Clinical Practice in human clinical trials
GPP	Good Publication Practice in professional medical writing
GRIPP	Guidance for Reporting Involvement of Patients and the Public in research
IER	Intervention Event Rate
MARS	Meta-Analytic Reporting Standards
MHRA	The UK Medicines and Healthcare products Regulatory Agency
OASPA	Open Access Scholarly Publishers Association
PRISMA	Preferred Reporting Items for Systematic Reviews and Meta-Analyses
RePAIR	Responsibilities of Publishers, Agencies, Institutions, and Researchers
RIAT	Restoring Invisible and Abandoned Trials

RIGHT	Reporting Items for practice Guidelines in HealThcare
ROBIS	Risk Of Bias In Systematic reviews
SPIRIT	Standard Protocol Items: Recommendations for Interventional Trials
TOP	Transparency and Openness Promotion guidelines
TIDieR	Template for Intervention Description and Replication
WHO	World Health Organization

1   *Introduction*

The pursuit of creating new knowledge enjoys a place of distinction globally. The public expects to reap benefits from scientific innovations. However, scandals of research fraud have shaken the trust that science once enjoyed in society. It is more important than ever that ethics and professionalism explicitly guide research integrity. Scientists are now expected to be more accountable than at any other time in history. Healthcare research is no exception. Academic institutions, funders, and journals are all under pressure. Have a look at the case study in Box 1.1.

Evidence-based medicine: The conscientious, explicit, and judicious use of current best research evidence in making healthcare decisions.

Evidence-based medicine can only work if it can deploy trustworthy evidence to inform healthcare decision-making and public policy. Behind modern medical interventions, there are many thousands of healthy volunteers and patients participating in clinical trials. It is these biomedical research studies that have led to breakthroughs in disease prevention and treatment in the last decades. The recent COVID-19 pandemic has shown how clinical trials have played a key role, particularly in national vaccination programs that helped bring societal restraints to an end. However, it is extraordinary that during the first four years of COVID-19 research, there had been over 400 retracted papers (retractionwatch.com, February 2024). This is a staggering number; nearly two papers were retracted per week. Just when the need for healthcare research was most important and urgent, society faced an avalanche of misinformation from scientists on a grand scale. In these cases, what happened to the system of oversight that research institutions, funders, and publishers were supposed to provide? Behind each of these retracted papers is a story of the failure of the stakeholder organizations in their role as guardians of research integrity. This background led to the idea of consolidating specific guidance on responsible clinical research conduct in this book.

Retraction: Removing a published paper from the research record due, for example, to the discovery of a flaw in its integrity.

Corrigendum: A correction notice concerning a published paper.

BOX 1.1: Case study – £1 million compensation after journal article retraction for research misconduct

- A pharmaceutical company sued a university for damages in a 2022 court case.
- One of the university's professors had undertaken research to evaluate the effects of a drug under contract with the pharmaceutical company and published a journal article based on the work in 2019.
- Concerns were raised about the published journal article on an academic online platform, and a corrigendum was issued in 2020.
- A research misconduct investigation took place at the university, and at its conclusion, the university wrote a letter to the journal.
- In 2021, the journal retracted the article, stating in its retraction notice that according

DOI: 10.1201/9781003461401-1

to the university's investigation, "misconduct did take place in relation to the research involved in this paper."

● The pharmaceutical company claimed in court that, as the paper had been retracted, the university was liable for breach of contract.

● In 2024, the court awarded £1 million in compensation.

Source: United Kingdom High Court Case number HT-2021-000478.
URL: www.bailii.org/ew/cases/EWHC/TCC/2024/35.html.
DOI: 10.1016/j.canlet.2019.05.028.

The research integrity focus of this book

Healthcare research is a vast scientific field. The corresponding research integrity field is accordingly vast as well. A large amount of pre-clinical or basic research is undertaken in laboratories, often involving animal experimentation. These findings inform what potential there might be in an intervention for helping humans. The scientific road from the bench to the bedside then takes its course through clinical trials (Box 1.2). Each step of this research translation journey has its own particular integrity concerns. Overall, in biomedicine, retractions are said to have quadrupled in the last two decades (DOI: 10.1038/d41586-024-01609-0).

The international recommendation documents or statements on research integrity consolidate concepts related to responsible research conduct broadly in science. Existing books on biomedical research integrity cover the topic in general. For example, they may state the importance of open science but may not specifically mention the research transparency elements required for integrity in randomized clinical trials. Transparency standards in such trials include open science practices such as prospective registration, protocol publication, *a priori* statistical analysis plans, data sharing, and timely and complete public reporting. The lack of specific guidance on randomized clinical trial integrity is a crucial barrier. This book addresses that gap.

Clinical trial: A prospective study of the effects of healthcare interventions. It may or may not involve random allocation.

Open science: An umbrella term covering various initiatives, such as prospective public research registration, open access publications, open peer review, open research data, and citizen science, that encourages sharing, cooperation, and knowledge dissemination without restrictions.

BOX 1.2: Trials covered in this book

A simple outline of research translation from bench to bedside in healthcare

	Pre-clinical research	Phase I	Phase IIa	Phase IIb	Phase III	Real-world trial	Phase IV
Bench to bedside	Laboratory research	Early translation		Late translation			Use in practice
Research type	Basic research				Applied research		
Clinical trial phase	Pre-clinical research	Phase I	Phase IIa	Phase IIb	Phase III	Real-world trial	Phase IV
Participants	Non-human	Healthy volunteers	Patients				
Study nomenclature		Safety, tolerability, dose finding, proof-of-concept		Explanatory or pilot trial	Confirmatory trial	Pragmatic trial	Surveillance
Participant eligibility criteria				Narrowly defined	Close to target population	Healthcare setting	
Randomization				Randomized clinical trials			

The terminology (this is a brief overview; see glossary for details)
- **Research translation:** Moving from the laboratory bench to the patient's bedside.
- **Clinical trial:** Studies evaluating the effects of healthcare interventions. In drug development, trials encompass a range of designs from large randomized clinical trials of patients (phase III) to uncontrolled observations of a few healthy volunteers (phase I).
- **Proof-of-concept study:** A clinical trial undertaken as an early translational step (phase I/IIa) to inform "go/no-go" decisions about proceeding with future randomized clinical trials (phase IIb/III).

What is covered in this book

- **Randomized clinical trial:** A clinical trial involving the random allocation of human participants to intervention groups and their follow-up to examine differences in group outcomes. This book uses the term "trial" as a synonym for a randomized clinical trial. It covers all ethics committee-approved trials involving eligible human participants who have a disease or condition targeted by the intervention, and who have given informed consent to take part (see Box 1.1 for a trial outline). A subclassification of trials is as follows:
  - **Explanatory trial:** A randomized clinical trial conducted under ideal, highly controlled conditions to generate preliminary evidence on the efficacy and safety of an intervention among a small sample of carefully selected participants (phase IIb).
  - **Pilot trial:** A randomized clinical trial in miniature form to examine the coherence of the various elements of a planned large randomized clinical trial.
  - **Confirmatory trial:** A randomized clinical trial that generates evidence on the effectiveness of an intervention in a large sample of eligible participants closely matching the target population (phase III).

- **Pragmatic trial:** A large randomized clinical trial that generates evidence on the effectiveness of an intervention in a real-world healthcare setting for optimizing its use in practice (post-phase III).
  (Note: The vast majority of randomized clinical trials are unclassified; see Box 2.3.)

What is not covered in this book

Research on healthy volunteers, studies without randomization, and feasibility studies carried out during the design or planning stages of a randomized clinical trial are not covered in this book.

Sources: nihr.ac.uk/glossary; clinicaltrials.gov/study-basics/glossary; htaglossary.net.
The demarcations between various stages and terms tend not to be as clear-cut as depicted; see the glossary and text for explanations concerning the grey overlapping zones.

Randomized clinical trials

Clinical trials form an important part of research translation. They bring about breakthroughs in disease prevention and cure by providing the underpinning evidence for the effects of treatments used in modern healthcare.

A clinical trial is any research study that prospectively assigns human participants to one or more healthcare interventions to evaluate outcomes. Interventions include a range of treatments, such as drugs, biological products, surgeries, radiological procedures, devices, behavioral modifications, process-of-care changes, and preventive care. Clinical trial designs range from observations of a few healthy volunteers at one end to large randomized clinical trials of patients at the other. The idea is to generate new knowledge through basic research, which, when taken forward through applied research, has the possibility of improving healthcare outcomes. The research translation journey from the proverbial bench to the patient's bedside requires a bridge where promising interventions are tested for their effects on patients before being considered for widespread implementation in healthcare practice. Randomized clinical trials, the focus of this book, are this bridge.

Throughout this book, the term "trial" refers specifically to a randomized clinical trial. Such trials are research studies approved by human research ethics committees that randomly allocate eligible, consenting human participants to intervention groups and then follow them up to examine differences in group outcomes (Box 1.2). Pre-clinical discoveries mature into treatments for use in routine healthcare practice through trials. Trials are the route through which new treatments complete their final journey into healthcare, improving outcomes for patients and the

Trial: Refers to a **randomized clinical trial** involving the allocation of eligible, consenting human participants to intervention groups and their follow-up to compare group outcomes.

Drug regulatory approval: Involves clinical trials in various phases: phase I focuses on the safety of a potential intervention in a few healthy volunteers; phase II helps to define an intervention (IIa) and gathers preliminary evidence on whether it can work (IIb); phase III gathers evidence on the effectiveness of the intervention; and phase IV helps discover the optimal use of an approved intervention in practice.

public. Trials evaluate interventions for their effects after the early stages of research translation have demonstrated their potential benefit. Taking the development of new medicines as an example, randomized phase II and phase III clinical trials are required for drug regulatory approval. The majority of the trials take place outside the drug and device regulatory framework. Regulators provide guidance about trials to manufacturers as a part of the approval process. Details of drug trials undertaken for regulatory approval are not covered by this book. Clinicians invited to take part in trials by pharmaceutical companies will benefit from developing a greater understanding of trials through this book.

The integrity of randomized clinical trials

This book focuses on the integrity of randomized clinical trials. Evidence-based medicine recognizes trials as being at the top of the evidence hierarchy. The intricacies of ethical and professional trial conduct will be covered throughout the chapters of this book.

Trials collate and analyze data obtained from human participants who consent to take part as research subjects. Trial participants are typically patients; exceptions include preventive intervention trials, such as vaccine trials, where participants are healthy individuals. Participants make this donation voluntarily, without the expectation of personal benefit. Some trials have tens of thousands of consenting, eligible participants enrolled. Without the volunteerism of these individuals, who make sacrifices for the sake of research during the course of their own illness, trials could not take place. Once trials are completed and their results are known, many others afflicted by the same ailments will receive improved healthcare. In this way, society benefits from trials. There is no escaping the fact that failures in trial integrity are a failure of the trust placed in trials by participants and society.

Retractions and expressions of concern are on the rise in published literature. In the PubMed database, there were over 250 trial retractions and expressions of concern in the year 2022, whereas in the early nineties, there were only a few trial retractions annually (PubMed, searched February 2024). This entails risks to patients and public health that need to be addressed at the root cause. This is particularly concerning as databases often fail to signpost trial retractions, and evidence syntheses continue to deploy such papers, potentially negatively impacting clinical practice guidelines. Every trial with an integrity flaw that remains unretracted presents a looming danger to healthcare. Failure to conduct timely and competent investigations of misconduct allegations is an important consideration in this regard. A system overhaul is required to address the problem of untrustworthy trials.

Expression of concern: A note published by a journal to inform readers of the possibility of a concern about the integrity of a paper.

PubMed: A freely available interface of the general biomedical research database Medline, which contains citations with and without abstracts (ncbi.nlm.nih.gov/PubMed).

In the first four years of COVID-19 research, among the over 400 retracted COVID-19 papers, seven were randomized clinical trials (retractionwatch.com, February 2024). The rate of retraction of trials due to integrity failures is difficult to establish. In part, this is because misconduct investigations are yet to be optimized both in terms of timeliness and competence. Their findings are often confidential, and retraction notices tend to be opaque. Estimates of research misconduct range widely, even as high as 25–33%. More middle-of-the-road estimates suggest that around 1% of retractions are related to data falsification and fabrication. However, it is clear that what we see on the surface is just the tip of the iceberg. No doubt, future research will help establish the retraction rate more accurately.

Evidence synthesis: A general term describing a systematic approach to collating evidence for developing clinical practice guidelines and policies.

The stakeholder organizations

There are many stakeholders in a trial. Individual trialists work within a research ecosystem made up of many organizations, each of which has the responsibility for fostering research integrity. In the case of a trial retraction, every organization that should have served to protect integrity has to go through introspection. Behind every retraction, there is a tale of system failure. Journals failed in the integrity assessment of the trial manuscript they accepted for publication; institutions failed in governance and audit of the trial conducted under their umbrella; and funders failed in oversight of the trial they financed (this is not a complete list). Prevention is equally important: What specific mechanisms should the various stakeholders have in place to nip the evil in the bud? What is clear is that stakeholders in the research integrity ecosystem cannot afford to work in silos. The need for increased inter-stakeholder communication and harmonization is all too apparent.

Journal: An establishment composed of editors and other publishing staff who organize the peer review of trial manuscripts and their publication.

Many countries have little or no experience in conducting trials, and many others do not have a well-prepared healthcare infrastructure. Moreover, there is considerable heterogeneity in healthcare systems across countries. This variation may result in differences in many aspects of trials. The human research ethics committee review and the institutional approval process may vary. Other aspects of trial conduct, such as data and participant safety monitoring, as well as data analysis and reporting, may also vary. There is a need for harmonization of research regulatory laws between countries at different levels of development. As the value of multicenter, multi-country trials is being recognized, there have been calls for international coordination between institutions, funders, publishers, and other stakeholder organizations such as the charitable sector, professional societies representing healthcare providers, consumer organizations representing patients, the media, the drug and device industry, and others. What specific actions should various stakeholder

Institution: A clinical academic organization, for example, a university or a hospital, where trials take place. Institutions have primary responsibility for the ethical and professional conduct of their trials.

Funder: Organizations such as governmental agencies, philanthropists, research charities, and industries that provide funding for a trial under contract to an institution.

organizations take? This book addresses this question, focusing on the role of institutions, funders, and journals.

Education and training

The value of trials fundamentally depends on the integrity of the information produced and published. Nevertheless, in medicine and allied healthcare professions, undergraduate and postgraduate education and training generally fail to adequately cover trial integrity in their curricula. Trial retractions are not always due to deliberate scientific misconduct; faults in technique and unintentional errors play their part. In trials undertaken for regulatory approval, the manufacturers receive guidance and supervision from regulators; they must follow the advice of the regulators to get approval. Otherwise, they would not be able to get permission to sell their products in the healthcare market. Funders of trials also insist on supervision. The majority of trials fall outside of the regulated and funded research environment. In these cases, without the guidance offered by regulators and funders, trialists contribute to trials as investigators more with good faith than with clinical research skills. Institutions have a role in supporting the trialists who undertake trials under their umbrella. Trialists need to be trained in how to plan, conduct, and report trials with integrity. Honest errors have the potential to compromise trial integrity as much as misconduct. Education and training in trial integrity are essential curricular requirements going forward. This book addresses this unmet need.

Readership of this book

This book consolidates in one place the clinical research integrity principles and standards that pertain to the randomized clinical trial lifecycle. Whether you are a specialist trialist or a journal editor, an overview of trial integrity across its entire lifecycle will be useful for you. Perhaps you will one day be part of an investigation dealing with a research misconduct allegation, or you will be supporting a trialist colleague going through such an ordeal. Perhaps you have concerns about a published trial and wish to make a formal complaint, or you have received a complaint that you think should be investigated. Through this book, you will gain an understanding of how misconduct policies and procedures should be judiciously applied.

The guidance in this book is pitched at a level suitable for non-expert trialists. It is aimed at a readership of healthcare professionals, master's and doctoral level students undertaking courses in healthcare research, epidemiology, and statistics, authors planning to conduct and report trials, human research ethics committee members, and administrators

Regulator: A formal body set up for official approvals of medicines and devices, for example, the European Medicines Agency (EMA), the US Food and Drug Administration (FDA), and the UK Medicines and Healthcare Products Regulatory Agency (MHRA).

Trialist: An investigator who makes a contribution to a trial and is credited in the authorship or acknowledgment section of the published article.

Research integrity: Undertaking trials in accordance with ethical and professional principles and standards. Integrity failures may result from honest errors or deliberate misconduct.

Principle: A moral value that guides trialists' behavior or conduct.

Standard: A specification of the conduct that must be adhered to when participating in or carrying out trials.

responsible for the governance of human clinical research in universities and hospitals, as well as journal editors, peer reviewers, and other editorial staff. Written in as non-technical a language as possible, this book will also be useful for wider audiences, including clinicians who recruit patients into trials, pharmaceutical and medical device industry professionals, patients, carers, and public representatives who engage in trials, members of trial oversight committees, research governance officers, systematic reviewers, guideline writers, funders of randomized clinical trials, medical journalists and bloggers, and individuals involved in trial management.

Policy: A guideline or set of rules.

Procedure: Step-by-step instructions for implementing a policy.

Chapter 1: Introduction – Key points

What this book is about

- In evidence-based medicine, the randomized clinical trial is the queen of the evidence validity dominion; it is placed at the top of the hierarchy for assessing the effects of healthcare interventions.
- This book describes the research integrity principles and standards related to randomized clinical trials, with illustrative examples covering the entire trial lifecycle, from conception to post-publication.
- Key points summarized at the end of each chapter include:
  - Specific advice to trialists on open science and enhanced transparency in trial design, conduct, analysis, and reporting.
  - Specific actions for the various stakeholder organizations to support trialists and to fulfill their roles as custodians of research integrity.

2 *Randomized clinical trials*

Knowing what works in optimizing healthcare, and what doesn't work, requires research. Of all the various research designs possible, the randomized clinical trial is the lifeblood of the evidence deployed in evidence-based medicine. It is ranked at the top of the effectiveness evidence hierarchy for making the strongest possible recommendations for healthcare practice and policy. Randomized clinical trials are research studies approved by human research ethics committees. A two-arm trial involves randomly allocating eligible, consenting human subjects or participants to a new intervention group or a control group and following them up to compare the group outcomes. This chapter will cover the basic outline of randomized clinical trials and the critical appraisal of their features that determine their usefulness.

Trial: Throughout this book, the term "trial" refers to a randomized clinical trial involving random allocation of eligible, consenting human participants to intervention groups and their follow-up to compare group outcomes.

An outline of a basic trial design

Evidence-based medicine paradigm places randomized clinical trials at the top of the effectiveness evidence hierarchy. Box 2.1 provides an outline of a basic trial design that compares two interventions: Following the human research ethics committee approval, the trial protocol is publicly registered; eligible participants are invited to take part from a population for whom the proposed new intervention is intended; they are asked to give informed consent; they are randomly allocated to a group that will receive the new intervention or to a control intervention group; the groups are followed up to determine their outcomes; and the group outcomes are compared to assess the effect of the new intervention.

Evidence-based medicine: The conscientious, explicit, and judicious use of current best research evidence in making healthcare decisions. It ranks randomized clinical trials and their evidence syntheses at the top of the effectiveness evidence hierarchy.

The term "arm" is often used to refer to the trial participant group that receives a specific intervention according to the approved trial protocol. A two-arm trial compares two interventions, but there are many variations on the basic two-arm design. Multi-arm trials compare various interventions. This book bases its discourse on a two-arm trial design unless otherwise stated. When a trial is planned, the extent to which the new intervention can work is unknown. This uncertainty forms the fundamental ethical and scientific justification for the trial (Chapter 4). The control intervention is usually the standard of care for the condition targeted by the new intervention. In some circumstances, with proper ethical and scientific justification, a placebo or no intervention may serve as the control. Following randomization, the participants are followed up to measure their outcomes. Trial groups should be treated identically during follow-up, except for the difference in the allocated intervention.

DOI: 10.1201/9781003461401-2

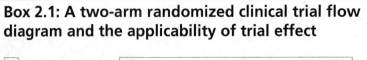

Box 2.1: A two-arm randomized clinical trial flow diagram and the applicability of trial effect

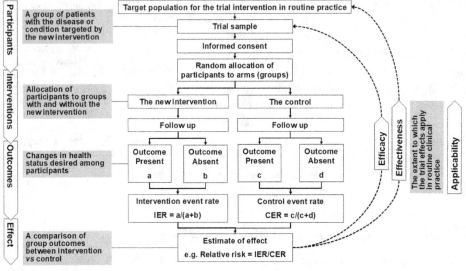

Trial components:

Participants: Patients or individuals with the disease or condition targeted by the trial intervention. Eligibility criteria are detailed, and those who meet all the inclusion criteria and none of the exclusion criteria are invited to take part. Trials may target healthy individuals for preventive interventions, such as vaccine trials or screening programs. Consenting, eligible participants are randomized.

Interventions: The new intervention could be a drug treatment, a medical or surgical device, a biological product, a radiological procedure, a psychological intervention, a process of care, a social or behavioral intervention, an educational intervention, a new vaccine, a preventive intervention, or a screening test. In a two-arm trial, it is compared to a control intervention, which is the usual care or the standard treatment for the disease or condition targeted by the new intervention. Both groups are treated identically except for the allocated interventions. In some circumstances, the control intervention could be a placebo or no intervention. Several interventions may be deployed in a multi-arm trial.

Outcomes: The changes expected in participants' health states, such as morbidity, and mortality. There may be various ways of measuring outcomes over different time horizons. The intervention groups are compared for differences in outcomes to estimate the effect.

Adapted from: DOI: 10.1201/9781003220039. Dashed lines: Applicability of trial effect.
There are many trial designs with different ways to recruit and randomize participants, to give them interventions, to follow them up, and to measure their outcomes. Arm refers to a group of consenting eligible trial participants receiving a specific intervention according to the approved trial protocol; a two-arm trial shown above compares the outcomes of two intervention groups.
Odds ratio is an effect measure for binary outcomes calculated as intervention odds (a/b) divided by control odds (c/d) (see Box 2.4); for continuous outcomes, the effect may calculate mean differences. For details of efficacy versus effectiveness see the relevant section in the text.

This is best achieved by keeping healthcare professionals and participants blind to the group allocation, if feasible. Outcomes are the health state or changes in the disease or condition targeted by the new intervention. The rates of the outcomes are computed per group, keeping the group composition fixed according to the initial randomized allocation. This allows testing of the trial's research question or hypothesis in line with its *a priori* statistical analysis plan (Chapter 5). The outcome rates are compared statistically to examine if the new intervention shows an effect in terms of improvement in outcomes relative to the control intervention group. The findings are transparently reported in a peer-reviewed journal as soon as feasible after trial completion (Chapter 7).

Randomized clinical trials are widely accepted as the gold standard for the scientific evaluation of intervention effectiveness in healthcare. This is because randomization helps create comparison groups that are similar at baseline with respect to the severity of the underlying disease or condition targeted by the trial intervention. When randomization is well-implemented, with concealment of random allocation sequence from healthcare professionals and participants in a sufficiently large trial, both known and unknown determinants of outcome, apart from the trial intervention, are likely to be distributed equally between the comparison groups. When this occurs, the groups are balanced for prognosis, or anticipated outcome, at baseline. In the presence of baseline comparability, the differences in outcomes between groups can be attributed to the intervention. This increases confidence that the observed effect of the new intervention, compared to control, is likely to be close to the "true" effect in the trial participant sample. In other words, this result is likely to be free of bias, or valid. In addition to concealed randomization, other trial design features, such as blinding healthcare professionals and participants during follow-up and at the time of outcome measurement, are known to help avoid or reduce the risk of various biases.

Validity and precision of trials

Trials should be designed to avoid or reduce the risk of two types of basic errors: systematic error, or bias, which refers to the tendency for the trial effect to depart systematically, either lower or higher, from the "true" result; and random error, which refers to the tendency for trials to produce unreliable or imprecise effects due to the play of chance.

The validity of a trial refers to the extent to which its results are free of bias within the participant sample. It is also known as internal validity, as opposed to external validity, which pertains to the applicability of the results among those targeted by the new intervention in the healthcare setting. To avoid confusion, this book uses the term "validity" to imply internal validity, referring to the risk of bias as a clarifier as required. It uses the term "applicability" instead of external validity wherever feasible.

Effect: The statistic that captures the observed association between interventions and outcomes (Box 2.1). It has a point estimate and a confidence interval.

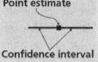

Point estimate

Confidence interval

Systematic error (bias): The invalidation of the observed trial effect due to weaknesses in trial methodology. Bias is distinct from research integrity flaws (Chapter 3).

Validity (internal): The degree to which the effect of the trial intervention is likely to approximate the "truth" for the participants recruited in the trial sample, i.e., are the trial results free of bias?

Random error: The tendency in trials to produce unreliable or imprecise effects due to chance.

Precision of effect: Error in effect estimation due to the play of chance or imprecision, often linked to small sample sizes and scarcity of outcomes. Imprecision leads to wide confidence intervals.

Bias may either exaggerate or underestimate the "true" effect of the trial intervention. Box 2.2 outlines four key bias: selection bias, performance bias, measurement bias, and attrition bias. As explained above, the avoidance or reduction of selection bias is primarily responsible for the high-rank trials have in the evidence hierarchy. Randomization achieves this through random allocation sequence generation and concealment of that sequence. The allocation sequence is prepared by a random number generator using variable block sizes to make it unpredictable, and to balance the groups for the number of participants. Additionally, groups are balanced for known prognostic factors using a procedure called stratification, to ensure that participants in each intervention group are closely matched for their demographic characteristics and prognostic factors at baseline. More sophisticated methods, such as minimization, dynamically balance both numbers and prognostic factors per group. This procedure aims to avoid the imbalances in unknown and unmeasured prognostic features between groups, allowing one to confidently attribute differences in group outcomes to the trial intervention. This requires making the allocation sequence non-manipulable, which is achieved through the concealment of the random allocation sequence from healthcare professionals and participants. This is possible even if blinding is not possible after randomization, and is best achieved by using a third party to assign group allocation after confirming participant eligibility. Group allocation should be kept concealed until informed consent has been signed, and until the time of the intervention.

Performance bias may arise due to unintended interventions or co-interventions that are not part of the trial protocol. Measurement bias may arise, particularly if the outcomes are subjective. Blinding healthcare professionals and participants during follow-up and outcome measurement is important for preventing both performance and measurement bias. If too many participants drop out, withdraw, or experience data loss, attrition bias may arise. The intention-to-treat analysis, along with imputation of the missing outcome data, helps to deal with this problem. A trial conducted with control of bias will produce valid results. Note that the issue of internal validity is distinct from the issue of research integrity, which will be covered in Chapter 3.

The issue of trial precision is related to its statistical reliability. The intervention effect is calculated by comparing the groups for differences in outcomes. The effect may also be described as treatment effect, estimate of effect, effect measure, or effect size. Various statistical measures of effect capture the strength of the association between interventions and outcomes, including relative risk, odds ratio, risk difference, or number needed to treat for binary data. For continuous data, it could be the mean difference or standardized mean difference. For example, relative risk is calculated by dividing the outcome event rate in the new interven-

Intention-to-treat: An analysis where participants are analyzed according to their initial group allocation, regardless of whether they dropped out, or fully complied with the intervention or not. A true intention-to-treat analysis includes an outcome (whether observed or estimated) for all participants randomized.

Statistical power: The ability to statistically reject the null hypothesis when it is indeed false. Power is related to sample size and the number of outcomes in the comparison groups. The larger the sample size, the greater the power, the narrower the confidence interval around the effect of the intervention, and the lower the risk that a possible effect could be missed due to the play of chance.

Box 2.2: Key biases in randomized clinical trials

Type of bias	Methods to avoid bias and report transparently
Selection bias	
Systematic differences between groups in prognosis or responsiveness to treatment.	• Generation of allocation sequence using a random number generator with variable block sizes to make the sequence unpredictable, and to create groups of roughly equal numbers. Stratification balances groups for known prognostic factors at baseline, while minimization dynamically balances the groups for both numbers and prognostic factors simultaneously. • Concealment of the allocation sequence from healthcare professionals and participants (this can be done even in unblinded trials). • A table of baseline group comparison for demographic characteristics and prognostic variables. Chance imbalances are more likely in smaller trials.
Performance bias	
Systematic differences in care provided apart from the intervention being evaluated.	• Standardization of care protocol. • Blinding healthcare professionals and participants. • The table of co-interventions demonstrating the comparability of the groups.
Measurement bias	
Systematic differences between comparison groups in how outcomes are ascertained.	• Standardization of outcome measurements. • Blinding participants and outcome assessors.
Attrition bias	
Systematic differences between groups in losses to follow-up, dropouts, and withdrawals from the trial.	• Intention-to-treat analysis. • The trial flow chart of participant follow-up from randomization to outcome measurement, including numbers with descriptions of dropouts, withdrawals, and data losses.

Adapted from: DOI: 10.1201/9781003220039.
Note that bias is an issue distinct from research integrity flaw (Chapter 3).

tion group by the rate in the control group (Box 2.1). The effect statistic has a point estimate and an associated confidence interval. The point estimate captures the direction and magnitude of the effect, while the confidence interval gives the imprecision in the point estimate, i.e., the range within which the value of the effect can be expected to lie with a given degree of certainty, such as 95%. The width of the confidence interval is related to the sample size and the number of outcome events within the comparison groups. If there is a low event rate and the trial lacks a sufficiently large sample size, it will have wide confidence intervals, leaving statistical uncertainty in the trial effect. In this situation, the result will likely be statistically insignificant, making it difficult to rule out the play of chance. A negative finding here would not be the testimony of the absence of an effect. It would be undue extrapolation or spin if equivalence between groups is claimed based on a non-statistically significant difference in the presence of a wide confidence interval. Needless to say, larger trials are required for greater statistical power, a concept explained in greater detail in Box 5.2.

Trials that are well-designed, well-conducted, and properly analyzed yield valid (unbiased) and precise results. The trial effects apply to the participant sample enrolled. Trials should also be designed and implemented in a way that permits the generation of results applicable to routine practice. For the societal benefits of trials to be realized, the valid (unbiased) and precise trial effects should also apply outside the trial in the populations from which the participant samples are selected (Box 2.1). What is the correct trial methodology to achieve this? There are no universally agreed criteria consolidated in the literature. Moreover, the terminology used to describe trials and their results can be confusing. The next section attempts to clarify the terminology and touches on the related methodological issues.

Effectiveness *versus* efficacy

The terms effectiveness and efficacy are often used interchangeably. To avoid confusion, they should not be deployed as if they are synonymous. There are also sub-terminologies within these terms that can further confuse readers. Effectiveness generally refers to the extent to which an intervention produces a beneficial effect applicable in a routine healthcare setting. Sometimes, a distinction is made between effectiveness in patients and effectiveness in practice. These two ideas approximate to the designs referred to as confirmatory and pragmatic trials, respectively, in Box 1.2. Some texts use the term efficacy to imply effectiveness in patients, so readers should be vigilant about the potential for misunderstanding. Efficacy, as used throughout this book, is defined as the extent to which an intervention can produce a beneficial effect in an ideal, highly controlled setting. This idea approximates to the design referred to as the explanatory trial in Box 1.2. In other texts, the term theoretical efficacy may be used to capture the effects observed in highly controlled settings. In drug development, for regulatory approval, the term explanatory trial maps to a phase IIb clinical trial, and confirmatory trial maps to a phase III clinical trial. Whether or not a pragmatic trial is a phase IV

Applicability (generalizability, external validity): The extent to which the effects of the trial intervention can be expected to apply in routine clinical practice, specifically to those for whom the intervention is intended in practice but who did not participate in the trial.

Effectiveness: The extent to which an intervention produces a beneficial outcome in the routine setting. Sometimes, a distinction is made between effectiveness in patients (confirmatory trial) and effectiveness in practice (pragmatic trial).

Efficacy: The extent to which an intervention can produce a beneficial outcome in an ideal, highly controlled setting (explanatory trial).

Some literature may use the term efficacy to mean effectiveness in patients, reserving the term theoretical efficacy for effects observed in highly controlled settings.

clinical trial remains a matter of discussion. Regulators provide guidance on design and terminology to manufacturers. This book focuses on advising trialists who do not have the benefit of input from regulators.

Having clarified the definitions above, what are the design and methodological features that make for an efficacy or effectiveness trial? How can one distinguish between trial results that pertain to highly controlled settings and those that pertain to routine settings? Given the variation in definitions, it would not be a good idea to rely solely on what the authors say about their published trial results. Certain trial features may help determine whether the findings may be applicable to the population for whom the intervention is intended in real-world healthcare practice. These findings will be more useful in directly informing healthcare practice and policy. By assessing these features, readers can make judgments about whether they can infer effectiveness, without the need for relying on the terminology used by the authors. Key applicability features are integral to the trial components (Box 2.1). These are outlined below:

Participants: The extent to which the participant sample represents the target population and setting for the intended use of the intervention is important. Broad eligibility criteria and recruitment from multiple centersprovide reassurance that the trial results may extrapolate from the participant sample to the target population. There should not be too many exclusion criteria, as this limits applicability. Explanatory trials tend to have quite strict inclusion and exclusion criteria, rather than capturing the heterogeneity that may exist in real-world settings. The exclusion of potential participants with common comorbidities is a particular concern in this regard. For this reason, diversity and inclusion are often recommended as important methodological considerations in trial design. The diversity of the participant sample is increased by deploying multiple trial centers. Broad eligibility criteria and recruitment from multiple centers also align with the goal of enrolling large participant numbers, which is relevant for the precision of the results when patient-relevant outcomes with low event rates are deployed.

Interventions: Interventions being trialed should be delivered with the resources, expertise, and flexibility typical of real-world practice, as targeted for future use. Comparing the intervention to a placebo or no intervention is likely to depart from real-world settings, where treatment options are often available for the target condition. Effectiveness trials compare the new intervention with the contemporary standard of care, permitting an evaluation of the potential benefit in the target population. Ideally, healthcare professionals and participants will be blinded to which group an individual is assigned to. The comparison of the trial intervention with placebo or no intervention creates an artificial situation that may assist in demonstrating a stronger efficacy assessment. In drug regulatory approval, placebo-controlled trials may be mandated by

Regulator: A formal body established for official approvals of medicines and devices, such as the Food and Drug Administration (FDA) and the European Medicines Agency (EMA).

Target condition: The disease or condition targeted by the intervention for use in healthcare, once trials have proven effectiveness.

regulators in phase IIb trials, but increasingly phase III trials are moving toward active treatment comparisons.

Outcomes: The outcomes measured should capture what is relevant to the patient. The effect of the intervention should be evaluated in terms of improvement in outcomes over a time horizon consistent with the impact of the target condition on the patient's life. For example, in cancer trials, 5-year mortality is a common outcome measure. However, efficacy trials tend to focus on short-term changes that reflect how the target organs or physiological systems respond, in terms of reduction in laboratory data and symptom scores. These surrogate outcomes tend to be more abundant, permitting achievement of precision in the trial result with smaller participant numbers. Extrapolating from these to real-world settings is difficult. In some circumstances, where surrogate outcomes are established to correlate with key, sparse long-term outcomes, the assessment of effectiveness may be achieved with moderate sample sizes (Chapter 5).

Effect estimation: A further feature relates to the analysis of outcome data collected from the participant sample. To begin with, the trial sample should be representative of the population with the target condition to ensure the applicability of the estimated effect in the healthcare setting. An intention-to-treat analysis is undertaken according to participants' initial group allocation, regardless of whether they dropped out or fully complied with the intervention. A true intention-to-treat analysis includes an outcome (whether observed or estimated) for all participants. The bias-reducing potential of randomization can only be realized when all randomized are analyzed. Efficacy analyses tend to focus on the effect among those who fully comply with the intervention, taking their findings away from the real world. This approach, also called per-protocol analysis, involves creating a participant subset less likely to be influenced by factors that could dilute the trial effect, thus, enabling a stronger efficacy assessment. However, this is only as far as it can go; it cannot represent an effectiveness assessment. The intention-to-treat analysis offers a comparison of a healthcare policy deploying the new intervention with the control treatment policy, making it much closer to real-world conditions.

Pragmatism

Pragmatism refers to the extent to which trials can be anticipated to produce useful results that directly inform healthcare practice and policy. Pragmatism features are broadly the same as those described in the section above. Pragmatic clinical trials generate effectiveness evidence after an approval has been granted to an intervention that requires regulatory approval. The aim of evaluating whether an intervention is effective in

Surrogate outcome: A substitute for direct measures of changes in health state, such as morbidity or mortality. These include short-term physiological variables, such as blood pressure for stroke or blood sugar for diabetic complications.

Per-protocol analysis: An analysis that includes only participants who actually received the intervention. Those who dropped out, did not fully comply, discontinued the intervention, crossed over, or received alternative interventions are excluded.

Pragmatism: The extent to which trials can be expected to produce useful results that directly inform healthcare practice and policy.

real-world settings for optimal use in healthcare is not unique to drugs and devices covered by regulatory agencies; all interventions need to be addressed for their effectiveness this way.

It is important to recognize how the journey through the early stages of research translation generates new knowledge as proof of concept (Box 1.2). Basic laboratory research that creates new knowledge is motivated purely by curiosity. As we move towards late translation, we enter the arena of applied research, which seeks to determine how new knowledge can inform practice and policy. Applied research is motivated by the desire to be useful in bringing about change in the real-world healthcare settings. Pragmatism in trials, moving from efficacy to effectiveness evaluation, helps get closer to this objective.

Around 25,000–30,000 trials are published annually in the PubMed database (Box 2.3), which includes around 5,200 biomedical journals. According to the Scientific, Technical and Medical (STM) publishers report, there are around 48,000 journals globally, and of these, around a third (around 16,000) are biomedical journals. So, PubMed captures only a portion of all biomedical journals, meaning there are likely many more trials published in total. Averaging the PubMed trial counts over the last decade, around 75 trials have been published daily. Overall, according to the indexing terms, phase II and III trials constitute only a very small proportion of the total number of published trials. These are explanatory and confirmatory trials undertaken for drug regulatory approval. Pragmatic trials, according to the indexing term, also make up a small proportion of the total. The vast majority of the trials, even when allowing for some indexing errors, remain unclassified. With so many healthcare interventions apart from drugs, it would come as no surprise that the majority of trials are not labeled with regulatory clinical trial indexing terms. A small proportion of these unclassified trials may be financed by a funder. Experience from evidence syntheses shows that the bulk of trials take place without the guidance of regulators and funders, in an environment where trialists contribute to a trial as investigators more with good faith than with clinical research skills. It is these trials that form the bulk of the evidence deployed in evidence-based medicine.

Critical appraisal of trials

Evidence-based medicine relies on trials to answer questions about effectiveness. Publication of a trial in a peer-reviewed journal alone gives no guarantees whether its findings will be useful in the healthcare setting. Even though the process for peer review vetting and editorial curation used by journals for publishing trials is considered the best available, it is imperfect (Chapter 7). Thus, critical appraisal has been recommended as part and parcel of the evidence-based medicine paradigm for several

Basic research: Motivated by curiosity, basic research aims to generate new knowledge.

Applied research: Motivated by the desire to be solve real-world problems, applied research aims to provide solutions.

Journal: An establishment composed of editors and other publishing staff who organize the peer review of trial manuscripts and their publication.

Funder: Organizations such as governmental agencies, philanthropists, research charities, and industries that provide funding for a trial under contract to an institution.

PubMed: A freely available interface of the general biomedical research database Medline, which contains citations with and without abstracts (ncbi.nlm.nih.gov/PubMed).

Box 2.3: Annual citation counts of the various randomized clinical trial types in the PubMed database

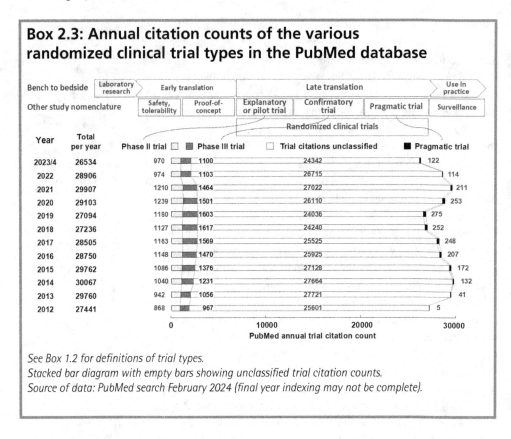

Year	Total per year	Phase II trial □ ▓ Phase III trial	Trial citations unclassified □	Pragmatic trial ▓
2023/4	26534	970 / 1100	24342	122
2022	28906	974 / 1103	26715	114
2021	29907	1210 / 1464	27022	211
2020	29103	1239 / 1501	26110	253
2019	27094	1180 / 1603	24036	275
2018	27236	1127 / 1617	24240	252
2017	28505	1163 / 1569	25525	248
2016	28750	1148 / 1470	25925	207
2015	29762	1086 / 1376	27128	172
2014	30067	1040 / 1231	27664	132
2013	29760	942 / 1056	27721	41
2012	27441	868 / 967	25601	5

PubMed annual trial citation count

See Box 1.2 for definitions of trial types.
Stacked bar diagram with empty bars showing unclassified trial citation counts.
Source of data: PubMed search February 2024 (final year indexing may not be complete).

decades. Existing critical appraisal guides typically seek answers to three simple questions asked in a fixed sequence: are the trial results: a) valid (unbiased); b) precise; and, c) applicable to patients? Progression is contingent upon positive answers at each step in the sequence. Otherwise, the trial cannot be considered useful for evidence-based practice.

To begin with, trial validity is the basic requirement for progression in the appraisal. If a trial fails on features of validity (internal), such as a high risk of bias on account of failures in the concealment of the allocation sequence from healthcare professionals and participants, any hope that its findings can be useful for practice is lost right there (Box 2.2). The next step, having established validity (internal), is the assessment of the precision of the trial effect. It will prove difficult for an imprecise trial effect, with wide confidence intervals, to come up useful. Should you throw out the valid (unbiased), imprecise trials at this appraisal step? This problem, in theory, may be dealt with by systematic reviews deploying meta-analyses.

Evidence synthesis: A general term describing a systematic approach to collating relevant evidence to address a research question.

Evidence syntheses of trials

Evidence syntheses of several small randomized clinical trials, with individual trial results statistically combined in meta-analyses, may produce effects with more precise overall results (Chapter 9). Metaphorically, this is the equivalent of turning noise into signal (Box 2.4). This concept is more easily understood by examining the graphical display of individual trial effects, known as a Forest plot. When using the odds ratio as the effect measure, the graph plots the x-axis on a log scale with a vertical line drawn at the value 1.0, which represents no effect, i.e., at this value, the odds of the outcome in the new intervention group are the same as those in the control group. For each trial, a box representing the point estimate of the effect lies in the middle of a horizontal line, which represents the confidence interval of the effect. The confidence interval is symmetrical around the point estimate. For outcomes that patients and practitioners wish to avoid, such as mortality, an odds ratio > 1.0 indicates that the new intervention is harmful, as the odds of death are higher compared with the control intervention. Conversely, an odds ratio < 1.0 indicates the intervention is beneficial compared to the control. A confidence interval that overlaps the vertical line of no effect represents a lack of statistically significant effect. When many statistically insignificant results are combined, the meta-analytic summary effect (usually presented as a diamond in the forest plot) may produce a significant finding.

Small trials may have been planned to address the intervention effect using a surrogate or composite outcome as the primary outcome (Box 5.2). The meta-analytic approach is particularly helpful when core outcomes are collected and reported in such trials, regardless of the primary outcome chosen for sample size estimation. For key core outcomes, when the overall confidence interval is narrower than in each of the individual trial results pooled in a meta-analysis, it is possible to move forward with the next stage of critical appraisal. Such evidence synthesis efforts may be useful for practice, subject to being able to meet some other methodological conditions such as a comprehensive search with

Systematic review: Summarizing the evidence using systematic and explicit methods to identify, select, and appraise relevant primary studies, and to extract, collate, and report their findings.

Meta-analysis: A statistical technique for combining (pooling) the results of multiple trials addressing the same question to produce a summary result.

Forest plot: A graphical display of individual trial effects, with 95% confidence intervals, in a systematic review along with the summary effect, if meta-analysis is used.

Corrigendum: A correction notice concerning a paper's version of record when the error(s) in the research work does not impact the main findings.

Box 2.4: Case study – Converting noise into a signal using meta-analysis

- During the coronavirus disease 2019 (COVID-19) pandemic, hydroxychloroquine, an antimalarial drug, was considered a possible treatment.
- Mortality is a core outcome for COVID-19 treatment trials.
- The trials ranged in sample size from 5 to 4,716.
- The trial results with respect to the effect on the mortality outcome made noise, rather

than sound. Due to the play of chance, none of the individual effects were sufficiently precise; the point estimates of the individual effects indicated the possibility of benefit (odds ratio < 1), harm (odds ratio > 1), or no effect (odds ratio ~ 1). Moreover, the confidence intervals were so wide around the individual point estimates that they always included the possibility of no effect on mortality (the odds ratio = 1).

- A 2021 meta-analysis combining the individual trials demonstrated that antimalarials were harmful: They increased the odds of death, with the entire width of the summary confidence interval above the odds ratio of 1.
- One of the included trials was retracted in 2022
- In a 2024 corrigendum of the original evidence synthesis, the updated meta-analysis, excluding the retracted trial, continued to show that antimalarials increase mortality (see Forest plot below).

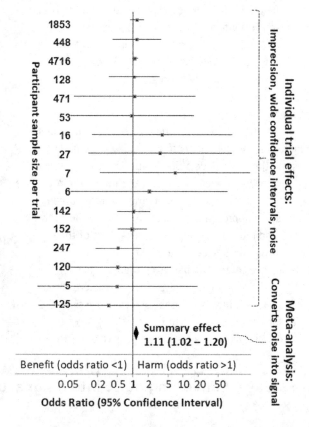

A Forest plot is a graphical display of individual trial effects (point estimates as boxes and confidence intervals as horizontal lines) along with the summary effect (diamond) if meta-analysis is deployed (note: in the graph above dimensions are not exact).
See Box 2.1 for an outline of a two-arm trial and calculation of the effect as odds ratio.
See Box 9.1 and 9.2 for definitions of evidence synthesis and related methods.
Sources: DOI's: 10.1038/s41467-021-22446-z; 10.1038/s41467-024-45360-6.

a low risk of missing trials, adequate trial quality, or low risk of bias. Valid (unbiased), small, imprecise trials may become useful when collated in evidence synthesis, especially when combined statistically in meta-analysis. If doubt remains after critical appraisal of meta-analyses, these evidence summaries may help as groundwork in the design of the large, effectiveness trials required. Frequently, well-conducted evidence syntheses conclude that more trials are needed. Thus, systematic reviews provide essential background to justify the need for a new trial in preparation for the trial protocol, both when seeking funding and when applying for human research ethics committee approval (Box 4.3).

The usefulness of trials

Historically, evidence-based medicine has focused primarily on examining the validity (risk of bias), precision, and applicability of trial findings. In trials with valid (unbiased) and precise results, critical appraisal typically ends by encouraging practitioners to ask: Are the results applicable to my patients? The results may appear applicable, but if they only capture surrogate markers and not patient-relevant outcomes, one cannot be certain about the usefulness of trial findings. Usefulness is linked to pragmatism, highlighting the distinction between effectiveness versus efficacy. It is important to go beyond the individual partitioner's perspective and ask more broadly: What is the extent to which randomized evidence with valid (unbiased) and precise answers can be useful for healthcare? The usefulness of trials is a multidimensional concept capturing more features than just the validity (risk of bias), precision, and applicability of findings.

For an intervention, once the preconditions of validity and precision have been met in an individual trial or established via a meta-analysis of trials at low risk of bias, the discussion about efficacy, effectiveness, and pragmatism can begin. An explanatory trial, undertaken with the intent of justifying a large confirmatory trial, provides the knowledge on which new trials can be based. In this sense, explanatory trials serve as proof of concept at the start of the late research translation stage. Their findings are useful for underpinning the protocols of confirmatory trials that will directly inform future practice and policy. However, efficacy evidence alone is much less useful for application to patients in the healthcare setting.

Box 2.5 builds on the outline of the research translation journey from bench to bedside, highlighting what makes randomized evidence useful. For trials to be useful, they should address an important societal problem. The importance of identifying research gaps and needs for determining trial priorities is covered in Chapter 4. Disease burden estimation is key, and both common conditions and uncommon conditions with major

Core outcomes set: A minimum set of critical and important outcomes on which there is consensus among patients and practitioners that they directly measure what is clinically relevant.

Research gap: A gap in knowledge.

Research need: A research gap that results in an inability to make healthcare decisions.

Composite outcome: A combination of two or more component outcomes into a composite. It may be difficult to interpret effects when comparing composite outcomes between groups.

Usefulness of trials: A multidimensional concept that evaluates integrity, research priority, pragmatism, validity, and precision.

Research priority: The ranking or selection of a few among the many established research gaps and needs.

quality-of-life impacts merit consideration for investment in trials. Once the priorities are established, trialists should aim for a trial setting as close to the real world as possible. Many confirmatory trials, while successful in paving the way forward, fall short of what is at stake in healthcare settings. A more pragmatic approach to trials is needed, rather than a more explanatory one, when an intervention has already passed the earlier stages of the research translation journey.

Moving towards the pragmatic end of the explanatory-pragmatic spectrum, participants invited to the trial should be similar to the patient groups targeted by the trial intervention in the healthcare setting. This is a key point, as the applicability of trial findings should drive the determination of the participants' eligibility criteria in trial design. This way it will be possible to extrapolate the trial results to those for whom the intervention trialed was originally intended, i.e., populations suffering from the target condition or disease during the course of their treatment in the healthcare setting. With overly narrow eligibility criteria, the evidence profile will reflect explanatory rather than pragmatic evidence. In addition to the liberal approach required in trial participant

Box 2.5: The relation between efficacy, effectiveness, and usefulness of randomized clinical trials

Bench to bedside	Laboratory research	Early translation		Late translation			Use in practice
Study nomenclature		Safety, tolerability, dose finding, proof-of-concept	Explanatory or pilot trial	Confirmatory trial	Pragmatic trial		Surveillance
Clinical trial phase	Pre-clinical research	Phase I	Phase IIa	Phase IIb	Phase III	Real-world trial	Phase IV
Randomization				Randomized clinical trials			
Trial effect type				Efficacy	—	Effectiveness	
Research integrity (trustworthiness)				Low transparency	—	High transparency	
Societal priority of the trial topic				Low disease burden	—	High disease burden	
Participant eligibility				Narrow criteria	—	Broad criteria	
Centre numbers				Single centre	—	Multicentre	
Comparison or control intervention				Placebo controlled	—	Standard care	
Outcomes				Low patient-relevance	—	Patient-relevant	
Outcome for sample size estimation				Surrogate (laboratory)	—	Core outcome	
Participant sample size				Small numbers	—	Large numbers	
Effect estimation				Per-protocol analysis	—	Intention-to-treat	

(Pragmatism features — left axis; Less clinically useful / More clinically useful — vertical axes)

See Box 1.2 for definitions of trials.
The demarcations between various stages and terms tend not to be as clear-cut as depicted; see glossary and text for explanations concerning the grey overlapping zones.
See Box 5.2 for sample size estimation.
See Box 9.6 for the usefulness of evidence syntheses of randomized clinical trials.
Source: DOI: 10.1111/1471-0528.17411.

sample selection, the choice of the control group plays a role. Patients and practitioners are interested in benefits that exceed the standard of care for the targeted disease or condition by the new intervention trialed. Therefore, if the control group intervention is placebo or no intervention, the trial results may not reflect the expected effectiveness of the new intervention in the healthcare setting. Statistical features also play a role in assessing usefulness. An adequately powered trial sould have a sufficient sample size to yield a precise result upon completion (Box 5.2). In this regard, the choice of the primary outcome measure is a key feature. The outcome should be patient-relevant and ideally selected from within a core outcome set, on which patients and practitioners have reached a consensus on regarding clinical relevance and importance. As explained above regarding effectiveness, the statistical analysis should follow the intention-to-treat principle.

The first spot in usefulness assessment, as outlined in Box 2.5, belongs to research integrity or trial trustworthiness. This book recommends that integrity assessment should be an independent item applied at the beginning of a trial's critical appraisal. A trial without integrity cannot be useful.

Research integrity: Undertaking trials in accordance with ethical and professional principles and standards. Integrity failures may result from honest errors or deliberate misconduct. Responsible research conduct paves the way for trial methods and findings to be regarded as trustworthy.

Critical appraisal: The evaluation of published evidence, whether trials or their systematic reviews, for their integrity, validity, precision, and usefulness.

The new trial critical appraisal

In the late 20th century, when critically reading papers, instead of blindly trusting the peer review process, emphasis was placed on institutional and journal reputations. Now, with institutions such as Harvard and Stanford under the cloud of research misconduct scandals (DOI's: 10.1038/d41586-024-00009-8; 10.1126/science.adj9568), and publishers, including top journal brands like Lancet and BMJ, under the burden of retractions (e.g., Box 10.5, DOI: 10.1136/bjsports-2022-106408), academic reputations are no longer the trustworthiness surrogate markers they once were.

This book puts research integrity first in the critical appraisal question sequence: Is the trial result: a) trustworthy, b) valid (unbiased), c) precise, and, d) useful? If a trial has integrity flaws, it cannot be useful, even if what is reported seems valid (unbiased) and precise. The question of trial trustworthiness should be raised by all readers of trials. This is measured by evaluating adherence to the open science standards of transparency (Chapter 7). It is particularly important for those with greater responsibility for critical appraisal, such as editors, peer-reviewers, systematic reviewers, and clinical guideline writers. Trial trustworthiness is the focus of this book.

Transparency in research: Open research practices, including prospective registration, protocol publication, a priori statistical analysis plan, data sharing, and timely and complete public reporting.

Planning trustworthy, useful trials

The usefulness appraisal outlined above (Box 2.5), you might be surprised to learn, has revealed that most published trials are useless for informing healthcare practice and policy. Not all valid (unbiased) and precise trials are equally useful; many are simply not fit for purpose. To this loss, you can add the burden of trials that are approved and commenced but never completed or reported. Coordinated campaigns, such as AllTrials and RIAT, aim to have all past and present trials publicly registered and correctly reported. Have a look at the case study in Box 2.6. The need for making extra efforts post-publication should be obviated by planning, conducting, and reporting trials with integrity in the first place.

AllTrials: A campaign for all past and present clinical trials to be registered, and their methods and summary results reported (alltrials.net).

RIAT: An international effort to restoring invisible and abandoned (unpublished and misreported) trials (restoringtrials.org).

This book argues that the motivation for trials should go beyond the desire for generating new publishable knowledge. The trial's clinical usefulness should be considered right from the outset when planning it, starting with the framing of the research question and the basic components of the trial design (Box 2.1). Explanatory trials may be valid (unbiased) and precise, but they are not directly useful for practice. To inform changes needed in practice and policy to benefit patients, trialists must make efforts above and beyond simply achieving validity and precision. Even when explanatory trials are strictly powered to generate efficacy data with small sample sizes and surrogate outcome measures, core outcome data can be secondarily collected and reported to allow useful evidence syntheses. Usefulness is not an optional extra; it is a fundamental ethical requirement for a trial's approval by the human research ethics committee.

Trials should be undertaken to generate knowledge that has the potential to inform healthcare decision-making, not just to "publish or perish" in academia. At the organizational level, institutions where trials take place and trial funders should seek a return on their investment in terms of usefulness, not just citation metrics. Journals should offer opportunities to publish all trustworthy randomized clinical trials, thoroughly discussing the extent to which the findings are clinically useful. This book aims to help both trialists and stakeholder organizations to deliver the most for society from the trials they engage in.

Box 2.6: Case study – A 2022 restoration of a 2017 trial

- A 2017 publication of a trial (registered in 2013) reported an apparent benefit of an intervention using a composite outcome measure in a trial that terminated early.
- A composite outcome, which combines several outcomes into a single measure, can offer increased statistical power, reducing the required sample size. However, the correlation that may exist between the components can lead to difficulties in the interpretation of the observed effect.

- The journal's correspondence section and online academic blogs commented on the paper. A 2019 comment that appeared on PubPeer, an online platform for post-publication peer review, stated: "By casting such a broad net, the investigators seem to be seeking evidence from any of the four elements in the so-called primary endpoint" (pubpeer.com/publications/61828207992EF360AEF89FCCFFE0F9).
- In the more detailed trial report submitted by the manufacturer for regulatory approval, among other things, the protocol with amendments, the outcome definitions and measurement, and the statistical analysis plan became available for re-analysis. These were obtained through laws governing public access to documents held by governmental agencies.
- It became possible to evaluate the causes of mortality that had not been previously reported.
- After independent re-adjudication of the outcomes, it was found that when the trial terminated early, there was a non-significant higher risk of cardiovascular mortality associated with the intervention.
- A complete restoration of the originally reported trial was recommended in 2022. On making the recommendation, the authors of the trial restoration stated that they had emailed the "editors to inquire whether they would be interested in learning about our RIAT project on the FOURIER trial, and also willing to correct the original article. In addition to the above-mentioned email, we also sent a reminder ... but never obtained any response".

See Box 5.2 for composite outcome measures and statistical power.
Source: DOI's: 10.1056/NEJMoa1615664; 10.1056/NEJMc1708587; 10.1136/bmjopen-2021-060172.
RIAT (Restoring Invisible and Abandoned Trials) restorations URL: restoringtrials.org/riat-studies.

Chapter 2: Randomized clinical trials – Key points

Execution of trials (advice to trialists):

- Plan trials for priority topics (Chapter 4).
- Frame research questions for trials defining participants, interventions, and outcomes with the usefulness of findings for practice in mind. Where this is not the case, ensure that the trial protocol, consent, and patient information pack explicitly refer to its preliminary nature.
- Design, conduct, and implement trials to produce valid (unbiased) and precise answers to the research questions, and report with transparency (Chapters 5–7).
- Set the trial in the context of existing evidence by undertaking evidence syntheses as part of trial panning. Keep the evidence syntheses initially undertaken updated throughout the trial and publish a definitive update on trial completion (Chapter 9).

TOP: Guidelines for Transparency and Openness Promotion (TOP) in journal policies and practices (osf.io/ud578).

Writing tips for trial authors:

- **Title page:** When using the term efficacy or effectiveness in the title, follow it with an explicit definition in the main manuscript text.
- **Abstract:** Ensure that the conclusion clearly states the extent of the clinical usefulness of the main trial findings.
- **Introduction:** Describe the trial's priority. Justify the trial in light of existing evidence synthesis (Box 4.3).
- **Methods, results, tables, and figures:** Follow research transparency principles and standards (Box 7.6). Thoroughly describe features related to integrity, validity (internal), and precision, ensuring complete descriptions of baseline characteristics, cointerventions, participant flow chart, and more (Chapters 5–7).
- **Discussion:** Include a full and honest discussion of the usefulness of the trial findings without spin. If the trial was preliminary, limit projections about the applicability of findings to planning future trials, not to healthcare practice or policy. Include an updated evidence synthesis, with meta-analysis if appropriate (Chapter 9). When recommending further research, give specific advice concerning the design and conduct of future trials.

Principle: A moral value for guiding trialists' behavior.

Standard: A specification of the behavior that must be adhered to when carrying out a trial.

Roles of institutions, funders, and journals

- Institutions, i.e., academic organizations such as universities and hospitals where trials take place, should encourage trials that are useful for healthcare, not just for creating new publishable knowledge.
- Funders that finance trials, such as governmental agencies, philanthropists, research charities, and industries should emphasize usefulness as a funding criterion.
- Journals should seek to publish trials with an explicit discussion of the clinical usefulness of the findings, recognizing that not all trials have the potential to inform practice or policy.

3   *Integrity of trials*

Recent admissions of questionable research practices and misconduct by the world's top academic institutions have undermined confidence in the trustworthiness of science. Beyond these headlines, research is an error-prone endeavor, and scientists are human. Research takes place in an ecosystem where scientists work within an organizational culture. Although organizations provide guidance for responsible research conduct, there are many grey areas in research ethics and practice. Organizational culture has a strong influence on researcher behavior. Scientists make judgments, and they may make innocent, honest mistakes. The extent to which these errors affect research integrity may go unscrutinized. Evidence-based medicine can only work if it deploys trustworthy research evidence to inform healthcare practices and policies. Randomized clinical trials, ranked highest in the evidence hierarchy, have come under the spotlight for having been retracted in large numbers following publication. Without integrity, any evidence, whether randomized or not, is useless. This chapter will provide an overview of what research integrity means and how it applies across the entire randomized clinical trial lifecycle, covering the role of trialists and stakeholder organizations.

Evidence-based medicine: The conscientious, explicit, and judicious use of current best research evidence in making healthcare decisions.

Research integrity: The responsible conduct of research in accordance with ethical and professional principles and standards. Integrity failures may result from honest errors or deliberate misconduct.

Responsible research conduct

The cat is out of the bag: there is no hiding the fact that scientists cheat. Recent admissions of questionable research practices and misconduct by academic institutions, along with large-scale retractions of published papers by journals, have undermined confidence in the trustworthiness of science.

There is no shortage of international statements and recommendations concerning research integrity. However, many fail even to attempt to give basic definitions. Research integrity is undoubtedly a broad concept. In this book, the term research integrity combines the notions of ethics and professionalism into an inseparable amalgam. Intertwining these two ideas allows the evaluation and oversight of a trial's conduct in light of established moral principles and professional standards. Following this definition, research integrity guidance can address ethical issues associated with randomized clinical trials and applicable standards, such as adherence to Good Clinical Practice in human clinical trials (GCP).

There are many terms and concepts to define and understand in the trial integrity discourse. To begin with, a principle is a value or concept that distinguishes between right and wrong and guides trialists' behavior. Taking the principles forward, standards specify the behavior that

Ethics: Decision-making based on moral values that distinguish between right and wrong.

Principle: A moral value that guides trialists' behavior.

Standard: A specification of the behavior that must be adhered to when carrying out a trial.

DOI: 10.1201/9781003461401-3

must be adhered to when carrying out trials. The aim is to help plan, conduct, and report trials in such a way that the methods and findings will be regarded as trustworthy.

Let's take, for example, the ethical principle of autonomy, which values the trial participants' right to make their own, independent, informed, and entirely voluntary decision to sign up for a trial. Several research conduct standards would apply at various stages in the trial lifecycle to ensure that trialists adhere to this principle. In the beginning, human research ethics committees ask trialists to use standard templates when preparing consent forms and patient information packs as a condition for granting approval to the trial protocol. During trial conduct, institutional research governance ensures that trialists implement the ethics committee-approved consent procedure in accordance to the GCP standard. To verify this, institutions might undertake research governance audits, which are planned formal evaluations of trial conduct, such as the review of its activities (e.g., observing the informed consent being obtained) and documents (e.g., checking that consent forms are correctly signed and dated, and securely stored). Finally, upon trial completion, when submitting the trial manuscript for publication, journals typically insist on reporting the details of the human research ethics committee approval in line with the guidance of the Committee on Publication Ethics (COPE). One might assume that researchers would automatically adhere to the integrity principle concerning respect for participants' autonomy and related standards, but this is not always the case. Unfortunately, there are many studies where they fall short. For example, a commentary on such a failure in a study conducted in the USA by its Public Health Service stated: "Despite 15 journal articles detailing the results ... informed consent was never sought" (DOI: 10.1164/rccm.202201-0136SO).

With this preamble, you can hopefully see that trialists have to engage with many stakeholders. Trials take place in institutions that have to meet the requirements of the national research regulatory laws. Trialists, who appear in the authorship or acknowledgements section of the published trials, are institutional employees. They should receive institutional support and oversight to foster research integrity in their trial work. This support should be harmonized across the research ecosystem which includes other stakeholders such as funders, journals, professional societies, consumer organizations representing patients, and others. This is the theory. The reality, however, is that the many stakeholder organizations involved each tend to have their own axe to grind. With little cooperation between stakeholders, there appears to be more noise than signal in the discourse about research integrity.

Institution: A clinical academic organization, such as a university or a hospital, where trials take place.

Research governance: The system set up by institutions to ensure that the conduct of trials under their auspices is in compliance with regulations.

Good Clinical Practice (GCP): A set of internationally recognized ethical and professional standards for the design, conduct, recording, and analysis of human clinical trials.

Journal: An establishment composed of editors and other publishing staff who organize peer review of trial manuscripts and their publication.

Committee on Publication Ethics (COPE): A committee that issues guidance to journals (publicationethics .org).

Intellectual honesty

How do healthcare researchers develop their sense of integrity? Certainly, early education and family values play a role in the shaping their ideas about honest behavior. Any integrity courses or the lack of such offerings in their education and training curricula must have an influence as well. In their professional life, the importance placed on responsible research conduct is probably influenced by many competing forces, including the trialists' internal moral compass, career ambitions, the reinforcement of integrity in their scientific discipline, the institutional academic incentive system, the awareness of the applicable research integrity policies, and the tolerance of questionable research practices and misconduct at the institutional workplace, to name a few.

Trialists' intellectual honesty, a scientific virtue or trait, is fundamental to the integrity of their work. Their good faith underpins the trustworthiness of trials. Traits such as an honest attitude, faithful performance of duties to adhere to standards, and an absence of intention to cheat are all implicit in the construct of intellectual honesty. The challenge is to plan, conduct, and report trials in a way that demonstrates this honesty. Open science initiatives, explained below, can help make intellectual honesty in trials explicit. For example, transparency in trial reporting to make methods, data, and analysis verifiable through practices such as prospective registration, protocol publication, posting consent form, and patient information pack publicly, *a priori* statistical analysis plan, and data sharing can help to lay it out in the open for all to see.

Funder: Organizations such as governmental agencies, philanthropists, research charities, and industries. that provide funding for a trial under contract with an institution.

Scientific virtue: A character trait or a disposition to function in a manner that will best achieve scientific excellence.

Misconduct: Unethical or unprofessional research conduct that is intentional, reckless, or negligent. Honest error is not considered misconduct.

Research integrity flaws

Failure of responsible research conduct is defined in two terms: questionable research practices and research misconduct. The definitions vary depending on jurisdiction (Box 10.2). Questionable practices and honest errors create an overlapping area between responsible conduct and intentional, knowing, or reckless misconduct. This is as far as the listings or definitions can go in classifying research conduct according to textbook theory. This approach views the problem of research integrity failure through the lens of misconduct investigations, which benefits from hindsight. In practice, however, there is a need to look prospectively at the issue of research integrity implementation, focusing the lens on the issues that arise as trials go through approval, participant enrollment, follow-up, data analysis, and reporting. There is a relatively large grey zone of ethical and professional dilemmas that trialists regularly face. Metaphorically, it represents the amber or red-orange signal between the red (stop) and the green (go) traffic lights; these dilemmas require judgment in the absence of specific guidance on whether to stop or proceed (Box 3.1).

Questionable research practices: Irresponsible research practices that are regarded as unethical or unprofessional but fall short of being considered misconduct.

Recklessness: Indifference or disregard toward the risk of producing false information from research.

Box 3.1: The relationship between various terms and practices related to responsible research conduct

Moral values A set of principles that differentiate right from wrong	Professional standard Specification of the behavior that must be adhered to	Research Culture The academic environment within research organizations

Responsible research conduct Compliance with ethical and professional principles and standards in the framework of the research culture

Trial design, planning, approval, conduct, oversight, analysis and reporting within the norms of the research culture

By-the-book responsible conduct (Green)	Grey areas requiring judgment (Amber)	Clearly irresponsible conduct (Red)
	Honest (unintentional) errors	Intentional, knowing or reckless

Research record creation via publication of papers in journals following editorial assessment and peer review

No integrity concerns	No concern raised	Integrity concerns raised			No concern raised
			Investigation		
		No case to answer	Questionable research practices		
			Research Misconduct		
			Research record correction		

The traffic light analogy puts responsible (green) and irresponsible (red) research conduct on either side of the dilemmas that require the use of researcher judgment in the absence of guidance (amber); integrity concerns may arise at any time during research conduct or publication (Box 10.1); definitions of questionable research practices and research misconduct may overlap (Box 10.2); investigation procedures vary between jurisdictions (Box 10.4); the demarcations between various terms and practices are not as clearcut as that depicted; see Box 5.3 for an example of a grey area requiring judgment where pre-specification of the statistical analysis plan transparently addresses the integrity concerns related to p-hacking; the covered area of boxes is not proportional to the problem or issue size; see Glossary and relevant section of text for explanations.

The traffic light analogy places live research conduct in a different context from the retrospective nature of misconduct investigations. It becomes possible to see trialists working dutifully under guidance, with responsible conduct when observing the green light and irresponsible when breaking the red traffic light. The scrutiny of institutional research governance officers and journal staff, whose role is to monitor compliance with ethical and professional standards, is akin to that of a policeman or camera watching by the traffic light. Sometimes, however, there is no one manning the traffic light. This illustrates that research integrity is truly about doing the right thing when no one is watching. It also shows that research integrity is about institutions and journals not falling asleep when they are required to be on watch; ensuring compliance with integrity standards is only possible when you are present. However, one cannot be on watch all the time and there cannot be an explicit standard for every single scientific aspect. Thus, research integrity implementation

Audit: A planned formal evaluation of trial conduct, including activities (e.g., informed consent), and documents (e.g., data collection and recording), to independently determine if the trial is compliant with its approved protocol and meets professional standards such as Good Clinical Practice in human clinical trials (GCP).

requires the creation of a research culture or environment that facilitates doing the right thing, especially when no one is watching, and doing the best possible thing when there is no standard.

For research integrity issues covered by ethical and professional standards, compliance can be delivered as expected, subject to training and support given to trialists. To foster integrity, institutions have the responsibility to train the trialists and oversee their performance. Compliance can be measured if the right tools exist, and giving feedback on objectively measured performance against integrity standards is a common aim of research governance audits. The standards come from guidance documents such as GCP. There are times when a trialist may not find any specific guidance, and they can seek advice from the human research ethics committees, and research governance officers. There may also be times when neither documents nor experts can give guidance. As fallible humans, trialists face uncertainties in the process of designing, planning, conducting, analyzing, and reporting trials where there are no scientific norms, leaving them with no clear-cut solutions. For example, how should a trialist deal with a conflict between scientific value and personal interest? Declaring the conflict of interest is fine, but transparency alone as a step forward may only be a partial solution. The context in which such an issue arises may be all-important in figuring out the solution. Editors, peer reviewers, and other readers appraising a trial manuscript may not understand the context due to lack of exposure to the world outside their setting, for example, when a developed country journal assesses a trial conducted in a less developed country. A solution found in one setting may not be appropriate for another setting.

The standard definitions of questionable research practices and misconduct (Box 10.2) are not helpful when addressing the problem at the level of trialist intention. The fundamental matter in responsible research conduct is that honest errors are not misconduct. This corresponds to the notion that intellectual honesty is based on truthful intention. The keyword here is "intention". This is something that is recognized even in criminal law, as a distinction is made between manslaughter and murder. In countries that have capital punishment, nobody can be executed for manslaughter, as it is considered less culpable than murder. While this is an extreme example, it explains the situation well. A research integrity flaw resulting from an unintentional error cannot, therefore, be considered misconduct. Solving problems with the best of intentions, with care, caution, and attention, but without clear guidance, cannot become misconduct. Training plays an important role here. The extent to which research competence is inculcated through training should help reduce the opportunities for errors. Formulation of sanctions is a challenging part of misconduct investigations when allegations pointing towards research integrity flaws have been found (Box 10.3). Training should be

Conflicts of interest: A potential or perceived compromise in the objectivity or judgment of anyone involved in research and publication due to financial or personal (non-financial) interests. Failure to declare conflict of interest is considered research misconduct.

Research culture: The academic environment consisting of the norms, values, expectations, attitudes, and behaviors within research organizations. Academic freedom, collegiality, collaboration, equality and diversity, research integrity (ethics and professionalism), openness, and transparency are all features of the research culture.

an element of sanctions, where incompetence is identified as an issue. An important consideration for research integrity investigators is the determination of the contribution of the workplace culture in their assessments. The lessons learned from investigations can help bring about continuous improvements in the research culture.

Authorship in "publish or perish" culture

Take the example of the tension that the most basic scientific matter, like authorship, can create in a competitive academic culture. Intellectual honesty requires that authors truly meet the criteria for authorship. In this regard, the International Committee of Medical Journal Editors (ICMJE) has defined the criteria and one of these requires final approval of the version to be published (Box 8.1). Highly prolific authorship is defined as authors who publish one full paper every five days (more than 72 full papers annually). Those highly prolific authors who truly meet the criteria certainly deserve to be applauded and rewarded for their professional competence and performance. However, with thousands of scientists demonstrating hyperprolific publication outputs, one might legitimately wonder if this level of productivity is achievable. In a commentary on this subject, the hyperprolific authors interviewed readily admitted to not meeting the ICMJE authorship criteria. The comment was made that "Not all authors had approved the final versions of their own papers, but all considered approval of the final version necessary for authorship" (DOI: 10.1038/d41586-018-06185-8). Thus, knowing that an authorship criterion is not met, scientists have been prepared to accept guest authorship (Box 8.3). This is not intellectual honesty. This is, as far as compliance with the ICMJE authorship criteria stands, unethical and professionally unjustified. Authorship abuse is classified as a form of research misconduct (Box 10.2). If no one is reprimanded, there would appear to be tolerance or acceptance of authorship abuse as a feature of high-level academic performance at the institutional level.

The publish-or-perish academic culture, i.e., measuring research performance based on the number of publications and citations, is widely believed to be behind the phenomenon linking academic productivity with authorship abuse. This incentive system adds fuel to the fire of competition in the workplace. It catapults some into pole positions through possible authorship abuse, coercive citation practices, and gratuitous citation. In this environment, scientists appear to follow the narrative of their employers for their appointments, annual appraisals, and promotions; they prioritize institutional expectations over notions of personal intellectual honesty. Acceleration, i.e., producing as many papers and

Authorship: Gives credit to those who make a substantial contribution in the design, conduct, analysis, reporting, and other critical aspects of a published paper.

ICMJE: International Committee of Medical Journal Editors has defined the criteria for authorship (icmje.org).

Authorship abuse: Unethical practices in authorship, including naming authors not strictly based on contribution, such as guest authorship, which may be part of highly prolific authorship (Box 8.3).

h(Hirsh)-index: A popular statistic to measure scientific output taking account of citations. For example, an *h*-index of 5 means that the author has 5 published papers that have been cited 5 times or more.

Publish-or-perish: An academic culture in which research organizations value the number of papers rather than their quality, integrity, or impact.

citations as fast as possible, is a key feature of this culture. A more sensible institutional narrative would be based on assessing academic output by accounting for publication norms and seniority according to scientific disciplines, or giving credit for scientific integrity and quality over quantity. So far, there are no signs of a change in the academic productivity narrative at the institutional or funder level. A collective response with institutions, funders, and journals working together as stakeholder organizations, could emphasize transparency in specific research contributions, moving away from traditional authorship (Box 8.2). This example explains why research organizations have to take responsibility for the integrity culture they nurture. Intellectual honesty is hard for researchers to exercise in an academic culture that lacks integrity.

Shades of grey in intellectual honesty

Trialists do not act alone, nor can they alone be the sole custodians of the research integrity of trials. They navigate within their research culture, positioning themselves within the expected norms.

To further explore the impact of the academic culture, let us take the example of another integrity flaw: Data-related misconduct, i.e., data fabrication (making data up) or falsification (manipulating or omitting data), can be behind trial retractions. Intellectual honesty requires trialists to deploy only true data to publish true results. There may be a requirement to omit data or to manipulate them to protect the privacy of trial participants. Data deidentification, anonymization, or pseudonymization (the latter permits the reidentification of trial participants if required) is legally required in many jurisdictions. Data alteration here raises no integrity concern, except in cases where this is not done or not done well. The protection of participants' privacy is a key ethical obligation regarding the intellectual honesty of trialists. It is the alteration of data with the intention to change the trial results in a particular direction that is falsification or fabrication and it is this that is regarded as research misconduct (Box 10.2). Data and result integrity are at risk when there is external or internal pressure, whether real or imagined, in the work of trialists.

Unfortunately, pressures to alter data and results can challenge the intellectual honesty of trialists. On the one hand, there are commercial interests of a trial funder that may put trialists under external pressure to produce positive results. On the other hand, there may be internal pressure arising from the perception that negative findings are worthless, such as failure to publish in impactful journals which are usually looking to publish positive findings. If the institutional workplace culture and incentive system values journal impact factors over integrity, this can heighten internal pressure. In an extreme situation, a research

The Coalition for Advancing Research Assessment (CoARA): Commits to abandoning inappropriate uses of quantitative journal- and publication-based metrics (coara.eu).

The Declaration on Research Assessment (DORA): Emphasizes eliminating the use of journal-based metrics, and instead assessing research on its own merits (sfdora.org).

Retraction: The removal of a published paper from the research record due to, for example, the discovery of a flaw in its integrity.

Impact factor: A popular statistic for ranking journals in order of perceived importance. It is calculated as the mean number of citations per article in a year taking as denominator the total number of citable articles published in the previous two years in a given journal. *Trials*, an open-access journal, had a 2022 impact factor of 2.5, i.e., the citable articles it published in 2020 and 2021 were cited on average 2.5 times in 2022.

integrity-naive trialist may start a career in an integrity-poor academic culture. They may even grow in this career and develop their own notions of integrity within a false belief system. Here, for instance, the academic entrepreneurial culture may promote the protection of commercial funding (driven by the publication of positive findings in high impact factor journals) to underpin staff salaries over research integrity. If everyone turns a blind eye, and no one discourages anyone who engages in data or result alteration, it would not be difficult for the personal norms of the staff to fall in line with those of the workplace. The pressure to put food on one's table every day, and without other options for work available, what other course could such a trialist take? This question is left open for perusal. This example is not to provide an excuse for intellectual dishonesty; it is merely to shed light on the real situation on many academic grounds. It reinforces the fact that the responsibility for the research culture at the workplace lies with stakeholder organizations. They all should work together to reinforce the right narrative. If institutions, funders, and journals all uniformly insist on open science initiatives requiring, for example, prospective public research registration, and data sharing, valuing transparency over secrecy, this will deter data fabrication and falsification.

Blatant data alteration is one extreme shade of grey that spills over into irresponsible research conduct. Another shade of grey is the selective outcome reporting, which alters results by taking advantage of transparency gaps. Yet another shade of grey, p-hacking, which exploits prevalent scientific uncertainty about data analysis (see below), may imperceptibly mix with responsible research conduct. In all of these shades of grey, there is a prominent organizational role in fostering the right research culture.

Scientific uncertainty

Uncertainty is an inherent aspect of clinical research and all scientific inquiries. Additionally, there is a level of uncertainty embedded within the culture and practice of research. These are referred to as the grey areas in Box 3.1. The emergence of flaws in research integrity can be seen as a consequence of how researchers navigate these uncertainties. The integrity standards exist to create clear demarcations, reducing uncertainties.

To explore the role of uncertainties that exist in the grey zone, let us take, for example, the well-known bias against publishing negative findings which is embedded within the research culture. This leads journal editors and peer reviewers to prioritize statistically significant findings for publication. This also is a factor behind the phenomenon known as publication bias. Within the limits of integrity standards, researchers can deploy strategies to create an advantage for themselves in the competitive

Selective outcome reporting: A difference in the outcomes in a published trial compared to its ethics committee-approved protocol. Prospective registration encourages reporting of the result for the original primary outcome, even if it shows a statistically non-significant result on trial completion.

Publication bias: The likelihood of publication of a trial is related to the significance of its results.

research environment. In trials, historically there was no prospective registration requirement for the primary outcome measure, so selective outcome reporting was practiced and tolerated in the past. Now, this door is being shut via the 2005 ICMJE trial prospective registration directive, which serves as an integrity standard today. Its full implementation remains an aspiration (Chapter 5). However, even when fully implemented, it cannot completely eliminate the possibility of cherry-picking. The door remains open to a sophisticated form of p-hacking in the trial statistical analysis plan if the primary analysis to test the main hypothesis is not pre-specified in black and white (Box 5.3). Trialists face scientific uncertainties in this regard. The statistical methods, for example, those related to the imputation of missing data, are many. In the absence of an agreed statistical standard, they have room for maneuver, i.e., they are in a grey zone where they can exercise judgment. To meet the journals' preference to publish positive findings, they can present the optimal result using the benefit of hindsight after performing the primary analysis in multiple different statistical ways. This practice may be better controlled in the future as robust statistical standards develop, but for now, this remains a grey area where no strict standard exists. Greater transparency through pre-specification of the trial statistical analysis plan and its public registration is the next step for implementation in research and publication practice by institutions, funders, and journals.

Cherry-picking: Reporting particular data and results while omitting others, a practice associated with the performance of multiple statistical tests in a dataset (fishing expedition) until one of them turns up significant, for example, the p-value observed crosses the statistical significance threshold (p-hacking).

Subversion of randomization

Concealment of randomization until the time of delivering the intervention, i.e., preventing foreknowledge of the group allocation, is what avoids selection bias in trials. It is this that makes groups similar at baseline (Box 2.2), and it is this feature that makes trials the queen of the evidence hierarchy. Now, what if randomization is manipulated? Intellectual honesty requires that clinical investigators who agree to recruit patients in a trial, should truthfully adhere to the approved trial protocol. Their trial's design and methodology would have been approved by the human research ethics committee. Additionally, governance approval would have been given in their workplace. The trial protocol would require that the randomization sequence is kept concealed, until the informed consent has been obtained. Once group allocation has been revealed, at the correct point in time, the intervention assigned will be implemented. As the clinical investigator would have obtained participants' signed informed consent, for them to then not follow the trial protocol, would be irresponsible research conduct and a breach of the duty of care. This should be a matter for institutional research governance oversight. On trial completion, the trial paper should explicitly report compliance with randomization procedures, as this holds the key to trial validity (internal), which is something that should be made a requirement for trial reporting in journals.

Randomization is usually administered by a third party outside the influence of the clinical investigator, such as via a telephone or a secure online system. This is to help avoid the possibility of manipulation by caregivers. Although difficult to imagine in the current century, sealed opaque envelopes containing the group allocation are still deployed in trials. These are readily manipulable. For example, a caregiver can peek into the group allocation by opening them in advance or by putting the envelope against bright light such as in an X-ray viewer. This allows for the possibility that clinical investigators give their favorite intervention to their patients by deliberately selecting or discarding particular envelopes, thereby defeating the purpose of randomization. Such a study cannot be called randomized. Even if the option of manipulation is eliminated through a third-party randomization system, clinical investigators may ignore the group allocation and deliver the intervention they prefer as their patient's caregiver. The power to rationalize and control care can lead clinical investigators to become non-compliant with the trial protocol. This practice has no justification. In one example where the randomization was to restricted or liberal use of episiotomy, clinical investigators who favored the procedure used it 90% of the time regardless of the group allocation. This led trialists to perform a post hoc observational analysis evaluating whether clinical investigators' beliefs concerning episiotomy affected the outcome (CMAJ 1995;153:769-79). Subversion of randomization is a serious trial integrity failure, as it downgrades randomized clinical trials to a lower rank in the effectiveness evidence hierarchy.

The clinical research ecosystem

Both individual and organizational behaviors contribute to the probability of conducting trials with integrity. The examples given above, concerning authorship abuse, data alteration, cherry-picking (p-hacking), and subversion of randomization amply, demonstrate the interaction between individual researchers' intellectual honesty and the research integrity culture that moderates it.

There are many more stakeholder organizations apart from the trinity of institutions, funders, and journals. These include, among others, the charitable sector, professional societies representing healthcare providers, consumer organizations representing patients, the media, the drugs and devices industry, and more. Together, they form a relatively complex ecosystem. What does the development of research integrity culture at the organizational level entail? Obviously, the stakeholder entities are bound by national laws. Institutions where trials take place have to formally

---

Clinical investigator: Healthcare professionals who execute trials in clinical practice according to the approved protocol. Where a trial site has many clinical investigators, one of them serves as the site principal investigator.

Validity (internal): The degree to which the effect of the trial intervention is likely to approximate the "truth" for the participants recruited in the trial sample.

Selection bias: Systematic differences in prognosis or therapeutic response at baseline between trial groups. Randomization (with concealed allocation) of a large number of participants protects against this bias.

Societies: Non-profit organizations that seek to further a particular healthcare profession and the interests of their patients.

comply with the requirements of the human research regulatory laws. Journals have much freedom from formal regulation in the publication of their scientific content (Chapter 7). However, the publishing universe and the galaxy of biomedical journals within it are gigantic. According to the Scientific, Technical, and Medical (STM) publishers report, there are around 48,000 journals globally. Of these, around a third (around 16,000) are biomedical journals. PubMed only indexes around 5,200 biomedical journals. Recognizing the need for self-regulation publishers have set up advisory systems such as COPE, ICMJE, and the World Association of Medical Editors (WAME). Organizational aspirations and actions, that make up their culture, are also shaped by the belief system that comes with the entity's traditions and its experiences. For example, scandals of misconduct and retractions may influence how the affected institutions, funders, and journals might behave.

There are many national and international research integrity statements. However, one size certainly does not fit all when it comes to responsible research conduct. It is well-known that there are disciplinary differences in perceptions about research integrity. In this regard, the responsibility lies with organizations to move from the general to the specific. National and international research integrity directives and statements are by their nature distal, not proximal, to the local context, i.e., the microculture within faculties and departments cannot be affected directly by these. For example, the authorship construct has no uniformity across disciplines. Thus, it would be hard to give guidance that would apply universally. Healthcare research is vastly different from humanities and astronomy, for instance. Tailored, subject-specific policies and procedures will have a greater prospect of being considered relevant and thus they will be more likely to be adhered to. Appreciation of this interdisciplinary variation is particularly relevant to universities where healthcare researchers work alongside scientists in many other subjects.

Existing science integrity directives and statements require translation into specific policies about trial practice. Some clinical research integrity recommendations are provided in Box 3.2. The academic culture and incentive system are widely regarded as the key drivers of the research integrity culture in the clinical research ecosystem. Assessments undertaken for appointments, annual appraisals, and promotions should reward research integrity over citation-based metrics. Research funders follow these metrics as well, and this does nothing to help institutions reframe their policies and culture. An analysis of the highly prolific authorship above frames authorship abuse within the metrics-based academic incentive system. Changing this deeply rooted poor academic practice will require the cooperation of all stakeholder organizations. The competitive academic culture worldwide should play by healthy rules.

World Association of Medical Editors (WAME): Aims to improve editorial standards through self-regulation (wame.org).

PubMed: A freely available interface of the general biomedical database Medline, which contains citations with and without abstracts (ncbi.nlm.nih.gov/PubMed). It covers around 5200 journals, whereas it is estimated that there are 16,000 biomedical journals.

Policy: A guideline or set of rules.

Procedure: Step-by-step instructions for implementing a policy.

When it comes to the prevention of scientific fraud, organizations must have policies and procedures for handling research misconduct allegations, but ideally, they should have to use them only sparingly. Throughout a trial's lifecycle, there are many opportunities to prevent integrity flaws before a published trial is subjected to an expression of concern or retraction. Organizations should undertake root cause analyses, learn from their research misconduct investigations (Chapter 10), and continuously make efforts to improve their research culture. Strong, relevant research integrity policies to underpin the right culture should help prevent research integrity flaws. All stakeholder organizations must sing from the same hymn sheet, acting harmoniously and synergistically.

> **Expression of concern:** A note published by a journal to inform readers of a potential concern about the integrity of a paper.

Box 3.2: Some recommendations for fostering healthcare research integrity at the organizational level

Institutions (clinical academic organizations, e.g., a universities or hospitals where trials take place)
- Focus on developing a research environment that values research integrity the highest.
- Develop and implement programs for universal researcher training with updates in research integrity.
- Redesign training in robust scientific methods, putting methods such as research design and statistics in the context of responsible research conduct.
- Offer a research design service for planning robust trials.
- Establish a human research ethics committee with an audit of its compliance with research regulatory laws.
- Strengthen research integrity oversight through robust research governance.
- Provide a secure, non-manipulable data storage and sharing infrastructure compliant with data privacy laws.
- Collaborate in multicenter trials without compromising on research integrity.
- Redesign the academic incentive system to avoid pressure to publish or perish; reward meeting the standards of research integrity.
- Manage conflicts of interest, protecting researchers from unjustifiable external interference and coercion.
- Establish open science as the standard for research and publication practice.
- Collaborate with other stakeholder organizations to correct the research record through the prompt, robust investigation of misconduct allegations against researchers.

Funders (organizations like funding agencies, philanthropists, research charities, industry)
- Publicly provide declarations of conflicts of interest of grant reviewers and committee members.
- Collaborate in co-funding with other funders without compromising on research integrity.
- Evaluate proposals considering scientific methods and research integrity, prioritizing science for the sake of society over science just of publication, i.e., align funding priority with ethical priority.

- Monitor funded research for compliance with research integrity standards.
- Set mechanisms in place to prevent unjustifiable interference by the funder as well as by external influencers such as politicians, commercial partners, etc.
- Support open science and prevent authorship abuse through contractually bound publication requirements.
- Demand robust research integrity policies contractually from the institutions funded, including training for researchers in integrity, research governance, academic incentive system not based on citation metrics, and investigation of misconduct allegations amongst other requirements for responsible research conduct.
- Collaborate with other stakeholder organizations in the prompt, robust investigation of misconduct allegations against funded researchers as well as against grant reviewers and assessors.

Journals (establishments that organize assessments of trial manuscripts and their publication)
- Embed transparency throughout the publication process.
- Prioritize papers that meet integrity and quality standards; giving preference to positive findings over sound science encourages questionable research practices, for example, p-hacking, and is linked to publication bias.
- Encourage reproducibility; novelty is not everything.
- Strengthen editorial assessment and peer review through training in research integrity.
- Implement open peer review including declarations of conflicts of interests of reviewers and editors.
- Collaborate with institutions to correct the research record through prompt, robust investigation of misconduct allegations against authors, peer reviewers, and editors.

Other stakeholder organizations including the charitable sector, professional societies, consumer organizations representing patients, the media, the drugs and devices industry, etc. all have to play their own part within the research ecosystem to deliver trials with research integrity.
Sources: DOI's: 10.1057/s41599-021-00874-y; 10.1007/s11948-019-00094-3.

Open science in trials

Research integrity should be put center stage to restore trust in randomized clinical trials. This is easier said than done when the traditional competitive academic culture is that of secrecy and mutual distrust. Open science is an umbrella term covering various initiatives such as prospective public research registration, open access publications, open peer review, open research data, and citizen science, that encourage sharing, cooperation, and knowledge dissemination without restrictions.

Science, until recently, has been closed. Upon acceptance of a trial manuscript, trialists transferred the copyright to publishers and the published paper went behind a paywall. Thus, published trials were only accessible to those who could afford to pay for them. The public at large, and the even scientific community itself, could not access trial findings.

Open science: An umbrella term covering various initiatives like prospective public research registration, open access publications, open peer review, open research data, and citizen science, that encourage sharing, cooperation, and knowledge dissemination without restrictions.

Those who could penetrate the paywall received the papers, but scientific details and data were usually hidden inside an inaccessible black box, limiting the opportunities for replication and integrity evaluation. The open science metaphorical magic bullet, or collection of bullets, for achieving research integrity in trials is outlined in Box 3.3. Open science not only opens the door to the possibility of accessing trial methods and data at the time of publication (Chapter 7), but it also promises to make trials transparent throughout their life cycle (Chapter 6).

In trial publications, transparency through a set of open science practices can make methods, data, and analysis verifiable. Trials should have prospective registration on an open official registry (e.g., clinicaltrails. gov), public availability of the complete human research ethics committee approved trial protocol and an *a priori* statistical analysis plan, statements confirming trial protocol adherence or modifications, evidence of independent oversight, funding disclosures, conflicts of interests declarations, and sharing of deidentified raw data compliant with privacy laws along with provision of statistical code and output (Box 7.6). Transparency does not have to wait until publication. From inception to publication a trial has a long journey passing through the hands of many. Human research ethics committees, funding bodies, institutional governance, independent trial steering and data monitoring, statistical analysis planning, journal editorial and peer review assessments, to name a few steps along the way. All of these deliberations along the way ought to be publicly posted contemporaneously as part of open science, making trial integrity explicit from start to finish (Box 6.2).

Transparency in research: Open research practices, including prospective registration, adherence to trial design, *a priori* statistical analysis plan, data sharing, and timely and complete public reporting,.

Box 3.3: Open science vision for randomized clinical trials

Initiatives	Specific open science practices	Guidance and vision
Citizen science	● Patient and public involvement ● Priority setting ● Core outcome sets	● GRIPP - Guidance for Reporting Involvement of Patients and the Public in research (equator-network.org). ● ACTIVE – A framework for citizen involvement in evidence syntheses bringing Authors and Consumers Together Impacting on eVidencE (DOI: 10.1177/1355819619841647).
Research culture	● Open science and transparency	● CoARA – The Coalition for Advancing Research Assessment commits to abandoning inappropriate uses of quantitative journal- and publication-based metrics (coara.eu).

		• DORA – The Declaration on Research Assessment recognizes the need to improve the evaluations of researchers and their outputs, eliminating journal-based metrics (sfdora.org). • SCOPE – A framework for evaluating research responsibly (DOI: 10.26188/21919527.v1). • TOP – Transparency and Openness Promotion guidelines in journal policies and practices (osf.io/ud578). • RePAIR – Responsibilities of Publishers, Agencies, Institutions, and Researchers in protecting research integrity (DOI: 10.1186/ s41073-018-0055-1). • TRUST – Transparency of Research Underpinning Social Intervention Tiers Initiative for evaluating the implementation of TOP guidelines in journals (DOI: 10.1186/s41073-021-00112-8). • BOAI – Open access as a means to the equity, quality, usability, and sustainability of research (budapestopenaccessinitiative.org).
Timely open publication	• Prospective registration • Protocol publication • Statistical analysis plan preregistration • Preprints • Open data • Analytic code availability • Open access • Pre-review • Open peer review • Open reports • Post-publication peer review	• WHO Statement on public disclosure of trials – The main findings should be submitted for publication within 12 months and be openly published within 24 months of trial completion (DOI: 10.1371/journal.pmed.1001819. s001). • AllTrials – All past and present Trials should be registered and their methods and results reported (alltrials.net). • RIAT – An international effort to Restoring Invisible and Abandoned (unpublished and misreported) trials (restoringtrials.org). • ICMJE – Trials must be prospectively registered and provide a data sharing statement (icmje.org). • EQUATOR: A network for improving health research reporting. Trials benefit from SPIRIT: Standard Protocol Items: Recommendations for Interventional Trials; CONSORT: Consolidated Standards of Reporting Trials; GRIPP; TIDieR: Template for Intervention Description and Replication, etc. (equator -network.org).

Responsible contribution	• Contributorship • Conflict of interest declaration • Funding disclosure	• CRediT – Contributor Roles Taxonomy is a system for classifying the roles played by individual authors and those acknowledged in a trial publication (Box 8.2).

See Box 6.2 for a proposal for a trial's complete and contemporaneous public documentation.
See Box 7.6 for the specification of instructions to authors for journals to publish trials responsibly.
Source: DOI: 10.1371/journal.pbio.3002362.

Chapter 3: Integrity of trials – Key points

Execution of trials (advice to trialists)

• Practice intellectual honesty in all aspects of trial planning, conduct, analysis, and reporting.
• Follow ethical and professional principles and standards at all times.
• Make research integrity explicit, going above and beyond what is required as the minimum standard.

Roles of institutions, funders, journals, and other stakeholder organizations

• The stakeholder organizations responsible for fostering the integrity culture of the healthcare research ecosystem need to collaborate in harmonizing their contributions, i.e., sing from the same hymn sheet.
• Shape the right workplace culture via local policies that promote healthcare research integrity. See specific recommendations in Box 3.2.
• Make continuous trial integrity training a feature of healthcare research culture. Base the curriculum on the open science vision for trials outlined in Box 3.3.

4 Ethics committee approval and participant consent

Ethics is a basic pillar of research integrity. For human research to be ethical, it must protect individual participants and serve the interests of society as a whole. Trials, like any research project involving humans, must first pass through a human research ethics committee established under the umbrella of national research regulatory laws. All trials must have this approval, whether or not they receive commercial funding. The ethics committee, which includes lay members, has the expertise required to assess the ethical issues in trial proposals. It examines the trial's societal priority, its scientific justification, methodological soundness of its protocol, potential risks to participants including data and privacy issues, informed consent, the accompanying patient information, and more. This chapter is designed to help trialists prepare a strong application for ethics committee approval and to robustly implement consent procedures.

Research integrity: Conducting trials in accordance with ethical and professional principles and standards.

Ethics: Decision-making based on moral values that distinguish between right and wrong.

Background to human research ethics

The fundamental ethical principles of autonomy (respect, self-determination), beneficence (promote well-being), non-maleficence (doing no harm), and justice (fairness) are taught in health and allied subjects. The curricular focus of these courses tends to be on healthcare provision, not on research, and most likely not on trial ethics. How these principles apply in randomized clinical trials is at stake when seeking and granting ethics committee approval.

As is clear from Box 4.1, the key concern for a human research ethics committee is that in any proposed trial, a relatively small number of individuals (who accept the risks of participation) will be invited to take part, while the benefits will be intended for those who do not take part, i.e., the wider society. When patients are invited to enroll in a trial, those extending the invitation are healthcare professionals providing care. Thus, vulnerability and the danger of exploitation are apparent. Human research ethics committees must be reassured by trialists that all potential participants will be treated with respect, their human rights and welfare protected throughout the trial, including the safeguarding of their data and privacy.

To briefly outline the history of human research ethics, the voluntary nature of the consent of human participants, their ability to withdraw

Human research ethics committee or **Institutional Review Board (IRB)**, set up under national research regulatory laws, is tasked primarily with the responsibility of giving formal approval to a trial proposal and monitoring the ethical conduct of approved trials.

Trial: Throughout this book, the term "trial" refers to randomized clinical trials involving the random allocation of eligible, consenting human participants to intervention groups and their follow-up to compare group outcomes.

DOI: 10.1201/9781003461401-4

themselves from research without giving a reason, the need for research to address essential societal priorities, and the requirement for researcher training, were all enshrined in what is known as the Nuremberg Code, developed in 1949. The Declaration of Helsinki in 1964 and its subsequent revisions asserted the importance of informed consent and recognized that legitimate research could take place with participants unable to consent themselves (e.g., minors, those embroiled in an emergency or crisis or intensive care, those with mental illness), but with safeguards put in place to protect them. In such cases, informed permission must be obtained from a legally recognized representative, such as parents in the case of minors. These guidelines are constantly being updated.

Principle: A moral value to guide trialists' behavior.

Standard: A specification of the behavior that must be adhered to when carrying out a trial.

Despite these research ethics directives being in place, there have been many examples of blatant exploitation. One such example is the Tuskegee syphilis study in the USA, where participants were recruited without their consent. In a 2022 journal article on the trials' 50th anniversary, Tobin wrote: "Despite 15 journal articles detailing the results, no physician published a letter criticizing the Tuskegee study. Informed consent was never sought; instead, Public Health Service researchers deceived the men into believing they were receiving expert medical care" (DOI: 10.1164/rccm.202201-0136SO). At the time of writing this book, these articles remain in the literature without any formal expression of concern or retraction notices by journals. However, this matter is not just old history. For example, an article at the heart of a UK child vaccination scandal was retracted in 2010 because the institutional claims that the research had been "approved" by the local ethics committee were proven to be false on an independent investigation by the medical professional regulator (DOI: 10.1016/S0140-6736(10)60175-4; Box 10.5). In another recent example, a 2023 review of studies, including trials published by a French research institute, there were many irregularities in ethics committee approvals, leading to expressions of concern being issued by journals (DOI: 10.1186/s41073-023-00134-4).

Retraction: The removal of a published paper from the research record, for example, due to the discovery of a flaw in its integrity.

Expression of concern: A note published by a journal to inform readers of a potential concern about the integrity of a paper.

Box 4.1: Brief overview of human research ethics principles

Autonomy: Potential participants should make their own, independent, informed, and entirely voluntary decision to sign up for a trial. Trialists must provide them with intelligible, appropriate to their level of competency, and complete information about the trial. They must also ensure that participants, whether patients or citizens, are not lured or forced into trials against their will or interests. This is especially important for potential participants with diminished capacity (e.g., minors, those embroiled in an emergency or crisis or intensive care, those with mental illness) who cannot be exploited. Minorities should be appropriately protected as well, while ensuring that their right to participate is not violated.

Beneficence: Trials should be undertaken with societal benefit in mind, not for the personal promotion of the researcher or the commercial interest of manufacturers. While there may be advantages to some stakeholders, such as professional or commercial benefits for researchers or manufacturers, these secondary interests should never take precedence over the primary societal interest. Trialists must declare any conflicts of interest. Benefits for participants may also arise through the process of taking part in a trial, and these should be balanced against the potential risks.

Non-maleficence: This principle requires that potential risks to trial participants are balanced against the benefits to be gained from undertaking a trial. Any risks to participants must be conscientiously minimized in trial design and implementation. Human research ethics committees must thoroughly examine this aspect. Monitoring risks to trial participants is a key obligation of trialists, and for this reason, ethics committees should also provide instructions on monitoring arrangements. This role is undertaken by institutional research governance offices. Depending on the level of risk and trial complexity, additional independent oversight, such as independent data monitoring committee (Chapter 6), may be required by the ethics committees.

Justice: For the trial proposal to be fair, it must address a relevant societal priority, and its participants, who bear the risks, should come from the same population that is expected to benefit from the results of the completed trial. In addition to addressing priority, trialists should consider fairness in terms of eligibility criteria and the choice of location for conducting their trial. In this regard, diversity and inclusion are relevant for the applicability of trial findings to those for whom the intervention is intended. Exclusion criteria cannot be unjustifiably based on gender, race, minority group, or other characteristics protected by law. In multi-country trials, participants cannot be drawn from less developed settings where there is no prospect of realistically being able to deploy the interventions trialed.

This is a basic outline; the details of general ethics, medical ethics, bioethics, law, and other related subjects are not within the scope of this book.

Human research ethics committee

In the 21st century, human research ethics committees (referred to as "ethics committee" or "the committee" throughout this chapter) have their role in trial integrity firmly established and enshrined in law in most countries. Research regulatory laws require that institutions, i.e., clinical academic organizations such as universities, hospitals, and other medical research centers, assess and approve proposed trials before they are initiated and monitor them for ethical conduct. This requirement is differs from the need for hospitals and clinics to have ethics committees for addressing controversies in clinical care. The laws vary across jurisdictions.

Institution: A clinical academic organization, such as a university or a hospital, where trials take place.

Human research ethics committees are set up at the institutional level and consist of health and allied professionals, trialists, statisticians, patient and public representatives, and members with legal knowledge. Typically, trials undertaken at a single institution, also known as a trial site or center, are assessed by the local research ethics committees. To facilitate multicenter trials, some jurisdictions may have a centralized assessment and approval system. Trialists must seek this central approval first before approaching local or individual institutional research ethics committees. In multi-country trials, trialists have to seek approvals according to the requirements of each jurisdiction separately. In Europe, multi-country collaboration is facilitated such that the approval in one country is recognized by the other European Union member countries.

It goes without saying that trialists must prepare a scientifically sound trial proposal and fully comply with the requirements of the ethics committee. The committee will need to examine the trial's priority and methodological soundness, and may seek external expert advice on these matters. It will balance the potential risks to participants against the societal benefits of the trial, ensuring the protection of participants' rights and welfare, including safeguarding their data and privacy. It will examine the procedure for obtaining informed consent and the accompanying patient information. Ideally, the committee's role extends throughout the course of the trial, including monitoring compliance with the standards of ethical trial conduct. In many settings, this compliance monitoring role is undertaken by research governance offices established by institutions, separate from the ethics committees. Where such arrangements do not exist, trialists should provide periodic and final reports to the ethics committee.

Trialist: An investigator who contributes to a trial and is credited in the authorship or acknowledgment section of the published article.

Research governance: The system set up by institutions to oversee that the conduct of trials under their auspices comply with regulations.

The trial priority

The trial proposal must address a demonstrable societal priority to meet the ethical principle of justice. Participants cannot be invited to consent to take part in a trial where they accept risks merely to generate data for scientific publications; there must be a justifiable societal priority for the topic to be addressed by the proposed trial. Determining research gaps, needs, and priorities is a discipline in its own right. The key issues that should be covered when justifying a trial's priority include, among others: the disease burden (incidence, prevalence, economic cost, impact on quality of life); importance to stakeholders (patients, carers, practitioners, policymakers, etc.); and the research need (a knowledge gap that limits decision-making capability). These features contribute to the assessment of priority when there are many known research gaps.

Work undertaken to help establish a trial's priorities is often already published in peer-reviewed journals. Sometimes, this work is undertaken by the trialists themselves in the lead-up to the development of their trial proposal. This background information should be cited and explained in the application prepared for ethics committee approval. The research

Research priority: The ranking or selection of a few among the many established research gaps and needs.

Research gap: A gap in knowledge.

Research need: A research gap resulting in an inability to make healthcare decisions.

Box 4.2: Simplified description of some methods used for establishing trial priority

Disease burden studies: Descriptive epidemiology, the study of disease distribution in a specified population, helps determine how many people suffer from a disease or disorder by estimating incidence, prevalence, and other factors. Formal disease burden estimates capture the cost of illness to society in terms of economic burden, years of life lost to illness, and more.

Stakeholder engagement: Questionnaire surveys, groups or panel discussion (e.g., focus group), individual interviews, and other related techniques can be used to assess the importance of a trial topic to various stakeholders including patients, carers, practitioners, policymakers, and funders. These methods can also be adapted to determine whether there is equipoise or a lack of consensus among practitioners regarding the use of the intervention to be trialed.

Evidence synthesis: A systematic approach to collating relevant evidence to address a research question. The questions may be narrow or broad. Evidence syntheses may collate results of previous studies to demonstrate the safety of the intervention to be trialed and its potential for benefit. The systematic review, the queen of this research genre, summarizes all the available research evidence on a clearly formulated question, using explicit methods to identify, select, and appraise relevant studies, and to extract, collate, and report their findings. Traditionally such reviews address narrow questions, such as determining the harmful and beneficial effects of a single intervention. Broad questions, such as those about the effects of multiple interventions for the same disease or condition, may also be addressed in systematic reviews or in evidence syntheses called overviews or umbrella reviews. These may or may not deploy statistical syntheses. A mapping review is an evidence synthesis of an exploratory nature, undertaken to describe or map a research topic. These evidence syntheses are called scoping reviews when the purpose is to clarify key concepts. These different review types are helpful in identifying gaps in the literature for the scientific justification of a new trial. See Chapter 9 for details (Box 9.2 provides definitions).

Source: DOI: 10.1201/9781003220039.

---

methods used to address the issues relevant to justifying a trial's priority include both quantitative and qualitative (Box 4.2). Epidemiological methods help determine the disease burden, while questionnaire surveys and focus groups capture the importance to stakeholders. Evidence syntheses identify the knowledge gaps. These are just a few examples of the broad range of methods available.

Trial scientific justification and methodological soundness

The question of a trial's ethical justification is integrally linked to the scientific justification of the research question it aims to address. Trialists need to persuade the ethics committee that their proposed trial is defensible in scientific terms. In preparing this assessment, trialists should cover the usefulness features outlined in Chapter 2 (Box 2.5). If the possibility of obtaining a valid (unbiased) and precise answer to the question of effectiveness posed in a trial is low due to a lack of methodological rigor, there cannot be an ethical justification to proceed. Scientifically unsound trials are unethical. Full stop!

Taking a two-arm randomized clinical trial as an example (Box 2.1), the intervention being considered for examination of its effectiveness must be known to be biologically plausible and safe. This is something that should have been established for the intervention in question through the earlier phases of research translation. In drug development, for example, pre-clinical, first-in-human, and first-in-patient studies should first demonstrate both biological plausibility and safety (Box 1.2). The implausible interventions should be dropped well before considering a randomized clinical trial in participants with the targeted disease or condition. The same approach should apply to trials of interventions that do not require regulatory approval. When developing trial proposals for new, safe, and potentially beneficial interventions, it is important to rationally select comparators. In real-world healthcare, there are often many options available for the condition targeted by the intervention. A potential participant, as a patient, cannot simply be deprived of one of the reasonable options just so that they can be part of a placebo-controlled trial. Systematic reviews or umbrella reviews with broad questions can help cover the range of options available for a given disease or condition and the effectiveness evidence for each (Box 9.5). Potential participants, as patients, have the right to receive available interventions known to be effective (beneficence) as well as the right to avoid interventions known to be harmful (non-maleficence) before being invited to take part in a trial. When effective alternative options are unavailable, placebo or no-intervention controls can become justifiable.

It goes without saying that every trial proposal must clearly state a scientific objective or hypothesis concerning the selected intervention and its comparator. For the hypothesis to be justifiable, there should be a demonstrable lack of firm effectiveness evidence. Repetition without scientific justification would be unethical, as potential participants should be offered treatments already known to be effective. Evidence syntheses can explore the literature to map the evidence gaps (Box 4.3). The gaps may pertain to the amount (absence or scarcity) of effectiveness evidence associated with the intervention. Systematic reviews, with meta-analysis if required, may be used to demonstrate that existing literature contains either untrustworthy evidence with integrity flaws, poor-quality evidence with a high risk of bias, conflicting results with both positive and negative findings, or imprecision in results with

Usefulness of trials: A multidimensional concept, evaluating integrity, research priority, pragmatism, validity, and precision.

Precision of effect: Error in effect estimation due to the play of chance or imprecision is linked to small sample sizes. Imprecision leads to wide confidence intervals in the trial results.

Validity (internal): The degree to which the results of a trial are likely to approximate the "truth" for the participants recruited, i.e., being free of bias in its participant sample.

Effectiveness: The extent to which an intervention produces a beneficial outcome in the routine setting. Sometimes a distinction is made between effectiveness in patients and effectiveness in practice.

Efficacy: The extent to which an intervention can produce a beneficial outcome in an ideal, highly controlled setting.

quite wide confidence intervals incorporating the possibility of no effect (Chapter 9). There may be a justifiable need to replicate existing trials. For example, the previously evaluated effects of interventions may need reconfirmation in a different participant group. The evidence gap may pertain to limitations in the range of participant characteristics covered in the existing trials against the breadth of the eligibility criteria targeted by intervention in practice. Applying the trial findings in a different setting may require replication with some modification to the intervention. The effects reported may only pertain to surrogate, not patient-relevant, outcomes. Additionally, it may be necessary to demonstrate that there is clinical equipoise or lack of consensus about the effect of the intervention in question among practitioners. Equipoise may be demonstrated using stakeholder engagement methods asking professional groups to rank their treatment preferences (Box 3.2). It may also be demonstrated by audits showing variations in clinical practice patterns or by conflicting recommendations in existing guideline documents.

Target condition: The disease or condition targeted by the intervention for use in healthcare, after trials have proven effectiveness.

Equipoise (clinical equipoise): A state of uncertainty about the effect of an intervention.

Once a scientifically justifiable hypothesis has been presented, a study with a properly estimated sample size should be presented. Statistical power is calculated to have the prospect of obtaining a precise answer to the research question posed on trial completion, i.e., estimating an effect size with a sufficiently narrow confidence interval around the point

---

Box 4.3: An outline of possible trial scientific justifications

- No trial exists, but the proposed intervention has demonstrable biological plausibility for the target condition, with evidence of safety, tolerability, etc.
- Trials exist, but existing evidence is uncertain due to untrustworthiness (integrity flaws), poor quality (high risk of bias), conflicting results (both positive and negative effects), or imprecise effects on patient-relevant outcomes (quite wide confidence intervals incorporating the possibility of no effect).
- Trials need replication. For example, the previously evaluated trustworthy, high-quality, precise effects need reconfirmation in a different setting for a justifiable reason, or the intervention should be re-evaluated for implementation with a substantive modification, or effects on patient-relevant outcomes may need to be established.
- Trials exist, but there is uncertainty about intervention use among practitioners who deliver healthcare, such as lack of consensus about the effect of the intervention compared to the alternatives available, unnecessary sizable variations in clinical practice patterns across a geographical region, conflicting recommendations in existing guideline documents, and more.

Sources: DOI's: 10.1016/j.jclinepi.2017.12.026; 10.1016/j.jclinepi.2017.12.027.

estimate of the intervention's effect on a carefully chosen outcome. An unpowered trial would be wasteful, as it would not deliver a precise answer (Chapters 2 and 5). An overpowered trial would entail unnecessary risk, exposing additional participants numbers above the most appropriate sample size without justification. Thus, the estimation of the sample size for capturing a clinically relevant effect with enough precision is not just of scientific interest (Box 5.2), but an essential requirement for trial ethical justification. Only the most appropriate number, neither too few nor too many, should be asked to take part. Other methodological aspects, such as concealment of allocation and blinding, should also be emphasized to reassure the committee of the trial's validity in relation to the "truth" of the results. Restricting the discussion to trial precision, the plans for achieving the sample size required may have to be backed by feasibility evidence. In any stakeholder engagement work undertaken in the lead-up to the trial proposal, responses may have been sought about potential participants' willingness to participate in the trial. Data may also have been sought about participating center numbers, potential numbers of patients with the target condition per center, and practitioners' willingness to offer the trial to their patients. If there is a key funding requirement, such as in case of an expensive intervention, then offers of funds may have been made by a funding body or a manufacturer. All this information should be shared with the ethics committee, because if the trial were likely to be unfeasible, i.e., likely to fail to reach its target sample size, then there may be a case for seeking approval for a pilot trial instead. In a large-scale trial that is potentially doomed to failure from the start, inviting potential participants to consent is unethical, as it would offer them a false promise of a potential societal benefit in the future.

In explanatory trials, which are justifiably based on the randomization of much smaller sample sizes, the hypotheses differ from those in larger trials. Rather than delineating the effect of the intervention on patient-relevant outcomes, the focus in such trials may be on the study of mechanisms or the definition of the intervention, such as finding a suitable dose that is potentially efficacious and safe. The gained knowledge will help to determine whether or not to progress with further research on the proposed intervention, and the direction of travel applied research should take. Explanatory trials would not address the effectiveness of the intervention for future societal benefit. Here, the ethical justification would be on different grounds. The potential participants will hopefully contribute to societal benefit in the distant future on the basis that their participation in smaller trials will help decide whether or not to go forward with larger, definitive trials subsequently. Ethical approvals for pilot trials would follow similar reasoning. Explanatory and pilot trials may also contribute to evidence syntheses (Chapter 9), and are

Effect: The statistic capturing the observed association between interventions and outcomes. It has a point estimate and a confidence interval.

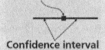

Pilot trial: A trial in miniature form to examine the coherence of the various elements of a planned large randomized clinical trial.

Explanatory trial: A trial conducted under ideal, highly controlled conditions to gather preliminary evidence on the efficacy and safety of an intervention among a small number of carefully selected participants.

Basic research: Motivated by curiosity, basic research aims to generate new knowledge.

Applied research: Motivated by the desire to be useful in solving real-world problems, applied research aims to provide solutions.

especially likely to be helpful if they collect and report core outcome data in addition to addressing their primary research question (Box 2.4). Being truthful about what can be gained from smaller trials is a key part of the patient information presented when obtaining informed consent. This is how small trials will meet the autonomy principle of research ethics.

Balancing the potential risks to participants against the benefits

The trial application to the ethics committee should justify the potential risks, and trialists should offer their assessment of how the benefits outweigh the risks. The main benefit is at the societal level, as future patients can receive better healthcare. The cohort of participants enrolled in the approved trial may also benefit compared to usual healthcare, as they may be able to receive greater medical attention by virtue of participating, such as through the vigilance of the additional staff employed for conducting the trial, the rigid protocolization of the healthcare they receive (whether or not they are allocated to intervention or control), and the independent safety monitoring implemented as part of the trial set-up. Risks involve exposing participants to the side effects of the new intervention being trialed. These risks must be balanced against the potential benefits by the ethics committee.

Healthcare interventions move from pre-clinical non-human research to research in healthy volunteers, and then to non-randomized trials in a selected subgroup of participants with the condition targeted by the intervention (Box 1.2). At each stage, more is known about intervention safety, tolerability, dose, and other basic biological characteristics. By the time a trialist prepares an ethics approval application for a randomized clinical trial, much is known about the potential risks to patients. During early research translation at each new stage, the risk is progressively reduced relative to the previous stage (Box 4.4). The risk is highest when intervention is first applied in humans, who are usually healthy volunteers. Next, the intervention is applied for the first time among a highly selected subgroup of participants with the disease or condition targeted by the intervention. Such studies require an extra level of care or vigilance. If the intervention causes substantial harm at any of these stages, its research journey is terminated early. The time for effectiveness trials is much further down the road. For example, in the case of drug development safety and dosing studies (phase I and IIa trials) are typically completed before the ethics committee application for a randomized clinical trial. Only those interventions that are reasonably low risk and show potential for benefit move on to being evaluated in trials. Examination of the effectiveness of the new intervention will often be in comparison to

Core outcomes set: A minimum set of critical and important outcomes on which there is consensus among patients and practitioners that they directly measure what is clinically relevant.

Participants: Individuals, also known as subjects, who meet the eligibility criteria and give informed consent to take part in a trial. In randomized clinical trials, participants are patients (with exceptions, such as preventive interventions like vaccine trials). Interventions target the disease or condition the participants suffer from.

Box 4.4: Conceptualizing the assessment of risk to participants in randomized clinical trials

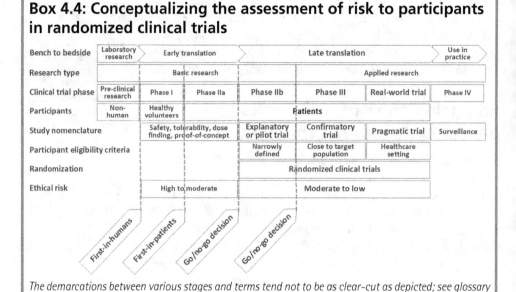

Bench to bedside	Laboratory research	Early translation		Late translation			Use in practice
Research type		Basic research			Applied research		
Clinical trial phase	Pre-clinical research	Phase I	Phase IIa	Phase IIb	Phase III	Real-world trial	Phase IV
Participants	Non-human	Healthy volunteers		Patients			
Study nomenclature		Safety, tolerability, dose finding, proof-of-concept		Explanatory or pilot trial	Confirmatory trial	Pragmatic trial	Surveillance
Participant eligibility criteria				Narrowly defined	Close to target population	Healthcare setting	
Randomization				Randomized clinical trials			
Ethical risk		High to moderate			Moderate to low		

First-in-humans   First-in-patients   Go/no-go decision   Go/no-go decision

The demarcations between various stages and terms tend not to be as clear-cut as depicted; see glossary and text for explanations concerning the grey overlapping zones.
See Box 1.2 for definitions of trials.

standard healthcare unless a placebo or no intervention can be justified. In this situation, by comparison to first-in-human studies, the level of risk is not as high.

Proper risk assessment of a trial proposal is best made when the details of all the previous research, whether or not published, are presented in the application made to the ethics committee. This is done ideally in the form of evidence synthesis (Chapter 9), such as a systematic review of the safety of the proposed intervention, included in the background section of the trial protocol with accompanying appendices describing the safety data in detail. The justification of the eligibility criteria outlining the characteristics of the participants who will be invited to participate should also be informed by a critical appraisal of previous research. There are inherent risks in the disease or condition targeted by the intervention. Both the intervention-related risks and the disease-related risks have to be considered. The latter is important for determining the control group, such as the level of disease-related risk may be higher under no treatment or placebo compared to standard healthcare. The degree of disease-related risk to participants in cancer trials may permit the committee to accept a particular level of risk of harm from the intervention to be trialed. By contrast, a benign condition will not permit acceptance of such an intervention-related risk. In specific circumstances, such as in younger participants compared to adults, or in pregnancy compared to non-pregnant individuals, the level of risk in particular subgroups may lead to their exclusion. Trialists should note that eligibility criteria assessment is important for ethics committees for several reasons. Beyond ensuring participant safety during the trial, eligibility criteria are directly linked to the applicability of the completed trial's findings among those for whom the intervention is intended in practice. The proposed trial when completed, must possess the potential to be clinically useful (Box 2.5). For example, if the intervention is intended for the elderly in practice, they must be included in the trial inclusion criteria with safeguards appropriate to their level of risk. Excluding them to minimize risk would limit the trial's applicability. The balance between risk to participants versus compromise in applicability is for trialists to explain and for ethics committees to evaluate. The trial usefulness feature is highly relevant to the ethical principle of justice.

The ethics committee would like to be reassured that participants enrolled in the trial will receive appropriate clinical monitoring and continuous attention to the protection of their rights and well-being throughout the trial. Ethics committee members may even be thinking about whether they or their own family members could safely join the proposed trial in making their judgment. To monitor risk during the course of the trial, an independent data monitoring committee (also known as the data and safety monitoring board) may be required by the ethics committee (Chapter 6). The monitors' deliberations based on the accumulating trial data may modify a trial's protocol or stop a trial during its course. This may require a confidential interim analysis. Trialists should anticipate the ethics committee's concerns in this regard, and proactively plan for safety monitoring. The ideal way to achieve this is through independent trial supervision (Box 6.1).

Participants' privacy protection is an obligation for trialists, not an optional extra. Data sharing is also increasingly becoming an obligation as part of open science. Many societal benefits are gained when data are shared. Compared to the culture of secrecy over data, sharing offers a level of transparency that serves to promote research integrity. The ability to independently replicate the results reported, undertake evidence syntheses with Individual Participant Data (IPD) meta-analyses, and perform secondary analyses after trial completion all add value to the case for approval by the ethics committee. In this regard, the informed consent and the accompanying patient information (see below) will need to cover key elements of privacy protection during data collection and sharing. The ethics committee would consider data collection and sharing plans as part of their risk versus benefit assessment.

Applicability (generalizability, external validity): The extent to which the effects of the trial intervention can be expected to apply in routine clinical practice, i.e., to those for whom the intervention is intended in practice but who did not participate in the trial.

Open science: An umbrella term covering various initiatives like prospective public research registration, open access publications, open peer review, open research data, citizen science, etc. that encourage sharing, cooperation, and knowledge dissemination without restrictions.

Individual Participant Data (IPD) meta-analysis: A statistical synthesis that uses participant-level data collected in the trials included in a systematic review to produce a powerful summary result.

The consent form and the accompanying patient information

The ethical principle of autonomy requires that informed consent is freely given. The ethics committee will examine this aspect of the trial proposal very carefully, as the potential participants' right to self-determination prevails over the interests of science and society. Informed consent can be considered "informed" only if it is accompanied by information giving details of the trial, the procedure for taking part, the risks and benefits, and so on (Box 4.5). If this background is not understood by a participant, the consent is not informed. The patient information sheet is the key document that the ethics committee will assess. It needs to be written in plain language, taking into account participants' level of education, familiarity with research, and cultural values. It may be accompanied by audio-visual aids. The consent does not have to be signed off in one sitting. The potential participants must have the opportunity to ask questions to help them develop a good understanding of the details. It is only then that they can make a voluntary decision.

When taking informed consent, special procedures are needed to help protect those who cannot protect their own interests, such as those who are mentally, physically, or legally incapable of making an informed decision. Children, for instance, will need their parents to consent on their behalf. Trialists should consider this issue within the justifiability of the eligibility criteria. Diversity and inclusion are relevant for the applicability of the completed trial's findings to those for whom the intervention is intended in practice. Exclusion criteria cannot be used to avoid the additional effort required to include participants with some incapacity. Participant characteristics such as age, gender, race, and minority group membership are protected by law. The ethics committee would want to ensure that inclusion criteria are as broad as possible, and that those with additional vulnerabilities are afforded additional protections. Scientific justification of the eligibility criteria should be linked directly to the hypothesis. For example, inclusion criteria may be narrowed down in case the trial objective addresses the efficacy of the intervention in question and vice versa broadened for addressing effectiveness. Limiting the inclusion criteria can hamper trial usefulness on its completion, impinging on the ethical principle of justice.

In certain circumstances, the need for obtaining consent may be waived by the committee. These are special circumstances and not the norm. The ethics committee would have to deliberate hard over this matter considering the practical feasibility of obtaining consent and the extent to which there would be an infringement of the ethical principle of autonomy in its absence. There must be strong justification on grounds

Equality and diversity: Diversity recognizes differences. People should not be disadvantaged because of differences in their gender, race, religion, disability, sexual orientation, and minority group membership (also known as protected characteristics).

of societal benefit in all such instances, with priority and scientific merit well established (the justice principle). The risk versus benefit argument should be strongly justified as well (the beneficence and non-maleficence principles). Then, the diseases or conditions for which consent exemption has been granted in previously published trials include life-threatening emergencies and critical illness, where it is impractical to obtain consent, but the family may still have the right on the patient's behalf to refuse participation. In cluster trials (undertaken in the real-world setting after confirmatory trials have already shown benefit), where communities are randomized to interventions, individuals within communities may not be approached for consent, but they may still exercise their right to refuse the intervention allocated to their community. In another trial design, consent may be sought only from those randomized to the intervention, not from those randomized to control, as they are allocated to receive standard healthcare that would have been provided in the absence of the trial. The waiver of consent is not a straightforward ethical decision. When seeking such a waiver, trialists must justify their request in consultation with and with the full endorsement of lay representatives of patients, carers, and the public. To meet all ethical requirements, it is far better to seek all the opportunities available to obtain informed consent than to avoid it. For example, in obstetric emergency trials, consent may be sought from all pregnant women at some stage during antenatal care, even though only a proportion may suffer the emergency for which the trial is designed for. In conclusion, requests for consent waivers for some or all of the trial participants should be sought with strong justification, only if alternative avenues have been explored and deemed unavailable.

Site principal investigator: The trialist or investigator coordinating all trial affairs in a trial site or center. There can be no trial without randomized participants who have complete follow-up data. This role is recognized in trial authorship or acknowledgment.

Shared decision-making is now a recognized requirement for ethical healthcare provision. The same applies when offering participation in a trial as an option to a patient. Disturbingly, as with consent for usual clinical care, evidence shows that research consent is associated with poor comprehension on the part of potential participants. Regardless of the comparison with usual healthcare practice, trialists have a responsibility to meet the ethical standards of research consent. How can the situation be improved remains an open question to be addressed. Audio-visual aids may help enhance the content of information shared for obtaining research consent, but technology has its limitations. Ultimately, there appears to be no shortcut to the time spent in face-to-face discussions with potential participants when it comes to ensuring their comprehension of what it would take to participate in a trial. This is the fundamental basis for fully informed, voluntary consent. Clinical investigators and research staff employed in trials as sub-investigators need training and protected time to achieve this objective.

Clinical investigator: Healthcare professionals who execute trials in clinical practice according to the approved protocol, including signing up trial participants and obtaining their informed consent.

Obtaining informed consent in a trial

Clinical investigators conduct trials on the shop floor, i.e., in the health-care setting. The process of obtaining informed consent in practice can only begin after the research governance department of their institution has formally given approval to commence recruitment using the ethics committee-approved trial protocol, consent forms, and patient information pack. In a multicenter trial, if central ethics approval has been granted, it must be ratified by the local institutional human research ethics committee as part of the governance approval. The timing of obtaining consent from the first participant is a key issue. It must wait until after the approved trial has been prospectively registered (Chapter 5).

Any licensed healthcare professional whose qualifications and experience permit the conduct and supervision of all aspects of the trial can be a clinical investigator. By law, healthcare professionals must be registered with a professional regulatory body to ensure that they are fit and licensed to practice. Thus dentists, doctors, midwives, nurses, pharmacists, physiotherapists, and other practitioners can serve as clinical investigators subject to the nature of the trial and the jurisdictional permissions. Depending on the trial, where many clinical investigators are involved, one of them may supervise the conduct of the trial as the site principal investigator. Sub-investigators may be appointed. All clinical investigators and sub-investigators would be bound contractually in employment. They will be required by the institutional research governance office to undertake verifiable trial training, such as Good Clinical Practice in human clinical trials (GCP), including periodic retraining during the trial's course. In some circumstances, the clinical investigator may have been part of the trialist team that designed the trial and obtained ethics approval of its protocol, but this is not a necessary requirement for taking up the clinical investigator role.

Many times, clinicians agree to participate in trials without fully recognizing the additional responsibilities they accept over and above their routine practice in doing so. The motivations for participating may vary, such as the desire for co-authorship (under the pressure to "publish or perish"), proving that their favorite intervention is effective, or financial compensation for themselves or their institution. In the case of funded trials, the funder would contractually bind the institution employing the clinical investigator. It is now important to recognize that without a proper understanding of their role, clinical investigators may end up subverting a trial. Chapter 3 covered this aspect with respect to the concealment of randomization and adherence to the intervention randomly assigned according to the approved trial protocol. Ethical and professional administration of informed consent in a trial is the most fundamental of the responsibilities of a clinical investigator. Specific consent training may

Good Clinical Practice (GCP): A set of internationally recognized ethical and professional standards for the design, conduct, recording, and analysis of human clinical trials.

Audit: A planned formal evaluation of trial conduct, including activities and documents, to independently determine if the trial (e.g., informed consent) is compliant with its approved protocol and meets professional standards such as Good Clinical Practice in human clinical trials (GCP).

Funder: Organizations such as governmental agencies, philanthropists, research charities, and industries that provide funding for a trial under contract to an institution.

Inspection: An audit conducted by an external legally competent authority.

Box 4.5: Trial participant information and informed consent basics

Content of the patient information package to accompany the informed consent:
- Trial title and summary.
- Contact details of chief investigator and site principal investigator.
- What will be involved in participation.
- What randomization entails.
- What if the potential participant declines to participate.
- The possible benefits and risks of participation.
- What happens in the event of an injury.
- Will any biological samples be retained.
- What if the participant wants to discontinue after signing up.
- How will participants be kept informed during the course of the trial.
- How will the participant's personal data and privacy be protected.
- How will trial data be prepared for sharing.
- How will trial results be shared with participants, if they wish to know.
- What treatment will be provided upon completion of the trial.

Format of consent:
- First contact information via poster, invitation email or letter, social media, websites, etc., prepared separately to trial patient information sheet.
- Plain language, co-produced with patient, carer, and public involvement.
- Keep the message neutral.
- Accompanied by audio-visual aids, mobile apps, etc., that are complementary to face-to-face contact.
- Time permitted for reflection.
- Opportunity to ask questions throughout the trial.
- Maintenance of confidentiality.
- Tailored to each setting in multicenter and multi-country trials.
- Consent training of clinical investigators.
- Clinical investigators as healthcare providers have power over patients which they cannot abuse to force them to enter into trials as participants.
- Audit by institutional research governance or external inspection.
- Update the information package, based on participant feedback or if new information emerges during the course of the trial. The updates need reapproval by the ethics committee.

The above is not a complete list; templates and requirements vary across jurisdictions. For transparency, it would be best to publicly post the unredacted consent form approved by the ethics committee without any personally identifiable information of the enrolled participants, e.g., with the trial registration or with the published trial protocol.

be formally required, in addition to the GCP certification, and this trial aspect may be subjected to institutional audit or external inspection for compliance with the approved protocol and standards during its course.

Focusing on obtaining informed consent correctly, it is not simply a matter of obtaining a signature on a form. Ethics committee approval and institutional research governance require that participants be fully informed about the trial. This is a process, not an act of signing the consent form. Potential participants must have the opportunity to learn about the trial to understand what they are being asked to sign up for. Consent is entirely voluntary. The information presented to them should be neutral and balanced. There should be no time pressure. Potential participants before formally enrolling in a trial should be given a copy of the patient information sheet to review in their own time. There may be an accompanying website or audio-visual material providing more explanation. They may discuss it with their close family, and they may be given the details of a clinical investigator who they can contact confidentially. With patient, carer, and public involvement, an independent citizen organization may help in the process of informing patients in lay terms. They may return to ask more questions before signing up or they may do so after having consented. They may not choose to participate once they understand the risks and benefits. They must be reassured that their care will not be affected if they decline to participate. If they choose to participate, it should be with full knowledge of what randomization entails; especially that they may be allocated to the control arm and that this is outside the purview of the clinical investigator. Once randomized, there is an obligation to follow up within the allocated group, until the outcome data are collected. In doing all this voluntarily, participants retain the right to discontinue for any reason or even without one, and this should not affect the healthcare they receive.

Power: The ability to influence others. The role asymmetry in a relationship permits the powerful to influence the vulnerable. The responsibility to prevent influence from turning into abuse lies with the powerful party.

Healthcare professionals are influential people. The power differential between them in their formal role as caregivers and their patients creates a level of vulnerability in the latter. This power differential arises due to the professional expertise, but also due to the expectations of the patients. The way healthcare professionals use their personal authority and power is relevant to obtaining informed consent for research from patients. It is always the responsibility of the healthcare professional to manage the risk of potential for abuse. They cannot force patients to enter into trials as participants. The decision must be informed and entirely voluntary. Occasionally, a patient as a potential participant or a signed-up participant may complain about the handling of the consent procedure. Instead of being put off, clinical investigators should participate in the handling of any complaints constructively in the same manner as would be expected of them in routine clinical practice. Participant feedback may lead to changes in the consent materials or procedures. If the information package or consent format is updated, this will require reapproval by the ethics committee.

Chapter 4: Ethics committee approval and participant consent – Key points

Execution of clinical trials (advice to trialists)

- Human research ethics committee approval must be obtained for all trials before potential participants are approached.
- Prepare the protocol according to the ethics committee's requirements. SPIRIT (spirit-statement.org) provides useful checklists for writing trial protocols (Box 5.1). Declare conflicts of interest in the protocol.
- Publicly register the approved trial on a recognized registry before starting recruitment, such as before obtaining consent from the first participant (Chapter 6). Include data sharing plans in the prospective registration.
- Publish the approved protocol in a peer-reviewed journal, whenever feasible.
- Prepare the consent materials and patient information pack truthfully with respect to the potential future societal benefits. Post publicly the unredacted consent form approved by the ethics committee without personal information identifiable. For example, append it along with the trial registration or the published protocol.
- Ensure that all trial staff are up to date with the training requirements, such as GCP certification and consent training.
- Implement the consent procedure with respect for participants' dignity and its voluntary nature. Clinical investigators should constructively take part in any complaints about trial consent procedures.
- Protect participants' confidentiality and privacy both in data collection during the trial's course and in data sharing following trial completion.
- Comply with research governance standards, actively taking part in any GCP audits and inspections. Establish independent trial steering and data monitoring committees taking into account trial complexity and risk (Chapter 6). The regulator, funder, sponsor, or ethics committee may mandate independent trial supervision.
- Report the main findings to the human research ethics committee on trial completion within 12 months.

Conflicts of interest: Potential or perceived compromise in the objectivity or judgment of a research ethics committee member due to financial or personal (non-financial) interests. Failure of declaration is considered research misconduct.

Regulator: A formal body established for official approvals of medicines and devices, such as the European Medicines Agency (EMA), and the US Food and Drug Administration (FDA).

Sponsor: Clinical trial regulations require that a sponsor makes proper arrangements to initiate and conduct trials. For trialists employed in an academic setting, it is usually their own institution that acts as the sponsor.

Writing tips for clinical trial authors

- **Title page and abstract:** Give trial registration details in line with the journal's instructions.
- **Introduction:** The trial justification, both ethical and scientific, should be provided as essential background.
- **Methods:** Human research ethics committee approval must be provided with the approval date. Give details of the consent procedures and justification for the use of standard care, no treatment or placebo as the comparator. Give information about participant safety monitoring, including details of any independent supervision given to the trial. Prepare a section on patient, carer, and public involvement, including its role in the consent materials and procedures. GRIPP checklist provides useful guidance for reporting citizen involvement.
- **Discussion:** Discuss the key ethical issues, especially the justification for any waivers or exemptions.
- **Acknowledgments:** Name independent members of the trial steering and data monitoring committees with their permission.
- **Supplementary material:** Signed and date-stamped human research ethics committee approval letters should be appended alongside the approved protocol including the consent forms and the accompanying patient information.

GRIPP: Guidance for Reporting Involvement of Patients and the Public.

Roles of institutions and journals

- Institutions should establish human research ethics committees and research governance offices according to the research regulatory laws. The legal details vary across jurisdictions. In general, the institutional responsibilities cover approval and monitoring of trials in compliance with ethical and professional principles and standards.
- The ethics committee membership should include lay representation. The membership should have the ability to assess ethical, methodological, and legal issues. The membership should publicly declare conflicts of interest (both financial and personal).
- The ethics committees should mandate that trialists prospectively register the trial with a data sharing plan before approaching participants for consent (Chapter 5).
- The ethics committee may, depending on the assessed level of the risk to participants, require trialists to establish independent trial steering and data monitoring committees for trial supervision as a condition of their approval (Chapter 6).

- Journals should mandate clear and explicit descriptions of ethics committee approval, informed consent and patient information, and the role of patients, carers, and the public in the development of consent materials and procedures in all trials (Chapter 7).
- Institutions and journals should cooperate in the investigation of allegations of ethical misconduct and consent irregularities, promptly issuing expressions of concern or retraction notices as required (Chapter 10).

5   Trial planning

DOI: 10.1201/9781003461401-5

Open science: An umbrella term covering various initiatives like open access publications, open peer review, open research data, citizen science, and more, that encourage sharing, cooperation, and knowledge dissemination without restrictions.

Transparency in research: Open research practices, including prospective registration, adherence to trial design, *a priori* statistical analysis plan, data sharing, and timely, complete public reporting.

Citizen science: An open science initiative encouraging public and consumer involvement in scientific research, with citizens actively making intellectual contributions.

Public documentation of trial plans at their start is now required as standard practice. The current minimum transparency standard is prospective registration, including a data sharing plan, before the first participant consents. However, this is insufficient for full transparency; the transparency principle should apply to other key elements of the trial blueprint. The unredacted, human research ethics committee-approved protocol, along with the consent form and accompanying patient information, should be published. Additionally, the *a priori* statistical analysis plan should be published unredacted before the trial database is locked. In fit-for-purpose trials, there will be citizen involvement with the aim of co-producing trials, with citizens co-authoring them. Patients, carers, and the public will take responsibility as co-investigators in trial planning, conduct and dissemination, instead of taking a passive part as trial participants or subjects. The conflicts of interest declarations of all trialists including the citizens taking part in trial co-production, should be publicly posted at the trial start and periodically updated. As well as patient, carer and public representatives, this chapter will give guidance to trialists, their institutions, funders, and journals on issues related to trial registration, protocol, and statistical analysis plan.

Patient, carer, and public involvement

Patient communities, carers, and the public at large are often unaware of the trials being planned, even though trials are meant to be undertaken for societal benefit. Paternalistic medicine is an outdated paradigm. A trial cannot simply be designed by trialists in their academic meeting rooms, isolated from the rest of society. Patient, carer, and public involvement is no longer an optional extra. Citizens should be partners in trial co-production, taking responsibility as co-investigators and co-authors for making their contribution (Chapter 8). They cannot just be participants taking part passively as trial subjects. It is now an old cliché that citizen science is research carried out with or by members of the lay public rather than being done about or for them, but it does capture the spirit of what is required in fit-for-purpose trials.

Patients, carers, and the public, representing those affected by or at risk for the relevant disease or condition targeted by the intervention proposed for the trial, should be invited to contribute early during the study design phase. Their input in defining the various trial components, such as participants, interventions, and outcomes (Box 2.1), is crucial to the relevance of the trial. They should remain engaged throughout the conduct of the trial as part of a strategy for maximizing research integrity. For a start, their role in producing easily accessible, understandable, and culturally appropriate patient information to accompany the consent form is an essential part of obtaining human research ethics committee approval (Chapter 4). Their contribution to improving the visibility of ongoing trials will help reduce the risk of recruitment failure. Their involvement throughout the course of the trial will aim to improve the protection of participants' rights and well-being. On trial completion, their efforts in dissemination will maximize the chance of trial findings becoming useful for healthcare.

So, what specific contribution can citizens make? Let us think through this in a logical manner. Obviously a trialist is not expecting a lay citizen to calculate the sample size and statistical power, although there could be rare exceptions when a patient representative may work as a statistics professor and may actually know how to do this calculation better than the trialists might. Well, this example is not to say that trialists should look for scientific expertise in their partnership with citizens; it is to highlight that citizen expertise may surprise trialists. Be prepared to be shocked and put the additional benefits acquired through the partnership with citizens to good use. This is a win-win situation!

The citizen contribution to trials can be continuous or sporadic in terms of involvement, and direct or indirect in terms of the method for giving input. The completed trial will inform shared decision-making between practitioners and patients in healthcare. Their opinion about trial priority is thus an essential input. Trialists may conduct questionnaire surveys, group or panel discussions, individual interviews, etc. with citizen to assess the importance of a trial topic (Box 4.2). When they undertake an evidence synthesis to map the evidence gaps, their citizen partners can be involved in the review formally opining on the literature collated. The priority established, citizens should be consulted in determining the acceptability of the planned trial to potential participants. This will make or break the trial. If patients do not accept the trial planned, there will be no participants recruited and there will be no trial. Even if, initially, patients can be persuaded to participate, in an unacceptable trial, there will be dropouts during follow-up, and without outcome data, there will not be any trial either. If there are doubts about trial acceptance among potential participants, it would be better to be less ambitious and undertake a pilot trial or incorporate an initial pilot phase within a full-blown trial. This approach, in case of failure to recruit the sample size estimated, will at least permit face-saving.

Which parts of trial design and conduct are best suited for citizen input? Trial priority establishment is a key citizen input regarding its justification (Chapter 4). Then, the assessment of participant eligibility criteria, intervention acceptance, and importance of outcomes are key citizen inputs to trial design (Box 2.1). In this regard, clarifying inclusion

Research priority: The ranking or selection of a few among the many established research gaps and needs.

Research gap: A gap in knowledge.

Research need: A research gap resulting in an inability to make healthcare decisions.

Authors and Consumers Together Impacting on eVidencE (ACTIVE): A framework for citizen involvement in evidence syntheses (DOI: 10.1177/135581961 9841647).

Participants: Individuals, also known as subjects, who meet the eligibility criteria and give informed consent for participating in a trial. In randomized clinical trials, participants are patients (exceptions include preventive interventions such as vaccine trials). Interventions target the disease or condition the participants suffer.

and exclusion criteria and their rationale in trials is one of the most fundamental aspects that will determine trial usefulness (Box 2.5). Eligibility criteria ought to consider both diversity, and representativeness of the participant sample with respect to the target condition. The intervention rationale, the related procedures, the mode of delivery, its frequency, duration, and intensity should be acceptable to patients. Some of this information becomes clear through the evidence syntheses undertaken in protocol preparation (Box 4.2), some through the real-world observations of clinical investigators in the trial sites that intend to take part, and some through the insights gained through the lived experience of patients involved as citizen representatives in trial co-production. A pilot trial could come to the rescue again if there is doubt about intervention acceptability. Intervention optimization could be a key step before launching a full-scale trial. In drug approval, this is achieved through early phase studies undertaken before launching a phase III trial. Core outcomes set development is a science in its own right. Trialists can initially shortlist outcomes of importance from a published core outcomes set they find feasible. They then can seek the prioritization of their citizen co-investigators to establish the primary outcome on which the trial will be statistically powered. Citizens as co-investigators providing the above input in trial co-production also play a key role in satisfying the requirements for human research ethical committee approval in providing input on the development of the informed consent procedures, forms, and patient information (Box 4.5). This way a truly patient-centered trial can be designed.

Citizen science is a part of the open science principles. If it is difficult for participants to locate the trial results, this may be because trial findings are not communicated to them in a timely manner or format. Citizens involved in trial co-production with trialists will be able to help in the dissemination of findings to participants and the community on trial completion more effectively than through publication in journals. They will also be able to persuade participants and influence decisions about data sharing, a key transparency aspect for enhancing integrity.

Pilot trial: A trial in miniature form that examines the coherence of the various elements of a planned large randomized clinical trial.

Usefulness of trials: A multidimensional concept, evaluating integrity, research priority, pragmatism, validity, and precision.

Target condition: The disease or condition targeted by the intervention for use in healthcare after trials have proven effectiveness.

Core outcomes set: A minimum set of critical and important outcomes on which there is consensus among patients and practitioners that they directly measure what is clinically relevant.

Box 5.1: Suggested trial protocol outline

Title page and front matter:
- Trial name, registration details, or plans (registration to be added after the ethics committee approval).
- Names, institutions, and affiliations of the trialists and citizens involved in trial co-production.
- Funding disclosures (direct support given by a funder for undertaking the trial).
- Version number and date (to easily recognize protocol modifications).

Background:
- The burden of the disease or condition targeted by the trial intervention and its research priority.
- Evidence of equipoise (the state of uncertainty about the intervention effect and its use in practice).
- Justification of the trial intervention and the comparator along with a description of potential risks versus benefits (give an evidence synthesis of the existing literature on the effects and safety of the interventions).
- Scientific objectives (framed as hypotheses concerning the effects of trial intervention).

Methods:
- Trial design (follow the specific SPIRIT reporting checklist that pertains to your design)
- Setting and participant eligibility criteria (keep the criteria sufficiently broad to help maximize the applicability of the intervention effect on trial completion in the healthcare setting; describe how sex, gender, and diversity-related issues have been addressed).
- Interventions (follow the TIDieR checklist to describe the intervention covering rationale, materials, procedures, competencies of the intervention provider, mode of delivery, the infrastructure required, the frequency, duration and intensity or dose, and acceptability to patients).
- Outcomes (select from the core outcome set relevant to capturing the effect of the intervention in terms of health improvement over a time horizon consistent with the impact of the disease or target condition on the sufferer's life, specifying the primary and secondary outcomes).
- Sample size (base it on the primary outcome measure) (Box 5.2).
- Recruitment timeline along with feasibility information.
- Randomization sequence generation, allocation concealment, blinding, and other related methods (give details of the random number generator used, how unpredictability is added via variable block size, what variables are used in stratification for creating groups balanced for key prognostic variables, if minimization is used how groups are dynamically balanced for numbers and prognosis, how allocation sequence is concealed, at what point the group allocation is revealed, and more).
- Data collection, recording, and management (including preparation for data sharing).
- Statistical methods (specify the primary analysis, i.e., the statistical methods to be applied to test the hypothesis concerning the intervention effect on the primary outcome; give the planned analysis for the secondary outcomes, subgroup analyses, e.g., those for sex and gender differences if appropriate, sensitivity analyses, etc.; confidential interim analysis plans for data monitoring if required).

Trial oversight:
- The trial steering committee and data monitoring committee.
- Planned research governance audits and any unannounced inspections.

Ethics and dissemination:
- Human research ethics committee approval or plan for seeking approval.
- Informed consent forms, patient information sheets, and other materials related to the procedure for obtaining consent (describing the involvement of the representatives of patients, carers, and the public).
- Dissemination plans (emphasizing open science in both scientific and lay outputs).

Other information:
- Declarations of conflicts of (financial and personal) interest of trialists, citizens involved in trial co-production, and independent members of trial steering and data monitoring committees.
- Case report forms (paper-based or electronic documents for data collection from the consenting participants).

The above pertains mainly to effectiveness trials and is not a complete list; protocol templates for ethics committee approval vary across jurisdictions; journals tend to follow SPIRIT reporting checklists.
Source: spirit-statement.org; tidierguide.org.

Trial protocol

The human research ethics committee reviews the trial protocol for assessment and approval. It should include the background of the target condition, the priority for the trial, an evidence synthesis of existing literature, the trial objectives, participants, interventions, outcomes, sample size and statistical analyses, methods, ethical considerations, dissemination plans, and more (Box 5.1). Sufficient detail should be provided to allow for appraisal of scientific and ethical issues. The first version of the protocol should be prepared according to the specific templates required as part of the application made to the ethics committee. This may or may not strictly follow the Standard Protocol Items Recommended for Interventional Trials (SPIRIT).

The trial protocol is a live document that may be revised during the ethics committee review. Trialists should register the trial prospectively according to the approved version of the trial protocol. Registration must happen before the first participant is enrolled. Then, it is recommended that the approved protocol be published. The protocol may continue to be revised following the ethics committee approval, registration, and publication. Substantial revisions will need further review and reapproval by the ethics committee. On trial completion, the last version of the protocol is usually submitted to the journal along with the manuscript. This allows journal editors and peer reviewers to assess the key methodological aspects in detail. They may ask for previous protocol versions to assess any changes that may have taken place. The last version of the protocol may also be provided as an appendix with the published trial. This helps others replicate the trial or to implement the intervention in practice.

EQUATOR: A network for improving health research reporting (equator-network.org). Trials protocols benefit from:

SPIRIT: Standard Protocol Items: Recommendations for Interventional Trials.

GRIPP: Guidance for Reporting Involvement of Patients and the Public.

SAGER: A checklist for gender-sensitive reporting.

DELTA: A checklist for reporting the sample size calculation in trials.

TIDieR: Template for Intervention Description and Replication.

Box 5.1 provides a suggested outline for a trial protocol. This serves as the tin or the container, while the content should take the form of a useful (Chapter 2) and ethical (Chapter 4) trial proposal. The background section of the protocol is the place where both scientific and ethical justifications are provided. This section should contain the trial priority based on disease burden studies (incidence, prevalence, economic cost, impact on life quality), the importance to stakeholders (patients, carers, practitioners, policymakers, and the public), and the research need (a knowledge gap, demonstrated through evidence syntheses, that limits decision-making capability). The trial scientific justification will seek to demonstrate that the trial intervention has biological plausibility and is potentially beneficial. An evidence synthesis should be included to demonstrate gaps (Chapter 9). The existing evidence may harbor integrity flaws, a high risk of bias, imprecise or conflicting results with positive and negative findings. There may be a demonstrable need for repetition, such as when the previously evaluated effects of interventions need reconfirmation in a different setting or with some modification to the intervention. The comparator will also need to be justified, especially if a placebo or no intervention control is used. Equipoise, the state of uncertainty among practitioners about the effect of the intervention, ought to be described (Chapter 4). This will underpin the scientific objectives and hypotheses.

The methods section of the protocol is where the potential usefulness of the trial on its completion is demonstrated. The protocol should permit the assessment of the applicability of the findings of the completed trial to the patient groups targeted by the intervention in the healthcare setting. The usefulness features require that the participant eligibility criteria are not narrow (e.g., taking sex and gender into account), that the intervention is fully described (using TIDieR checklist), and that the outcomes are relevant to patients (e.g., they cover the core outcomes set). The trial should be powered with enough sample size to have the possibility of delivering a sufficiently precise answer for addressing the question concerning the intervention effect on the primary outcome measure using intention-to-treat analysis (Box 5.2). There may be a tendency to deploy surrogate continuous outcomes or composite outcomes to reduce sample size requirements. Composite outcomes, combining two or more component outcomes, should be constructed soundly. The components of the composite outcome should be of a similar level of patient relevance, similar frequency of occurrence over the follow-up period, and similar in response to the intervention. Difficulties in interpretation may arise on trial completion using composites (Box 2.6). The trial feasibility information, such as potential participating numbers per center, potential patient numbers per center, practitioners' willingness to offer the trial to their patients, funding obtained to directly support the

Equipoise (clinical equipoise): State of uncertainty about the effect of an intervention.

Statistical power: The ability to statistically reject the null hypothesis when it is indeed false. Power is related to sample size and the number of outcomes in the comparison groups. The larger the sample size, the more the power, the narrower the confidence interval around the effect of the intervention, and the lower the risk that a possible effect could be missed due to the play of chance.

Composite outcome: Combination of two or more component outcomes into a composite. It may help reduce the sample size required. It may be difficult to interpret effects comparing composite outcomes between groups.

trial, etc. will reassure about the possibility of reaching the target sample size. Methodological details covering randomization sequence generation, allocation concealment, and blinding will ensure that the risk of various biases will be minimized. The establishment of independent oversight committees and engagement in research governance audits and inspections will ensure the conduct of the planned trial with integrity (Chapter 6).

Additional information should include details of the informed consent form, patient information sheet, case report forms, conflicts of interest declarations, and other relevant documents. As things develop further in the transparency arena, there is a real possibility that the informed consent form will be formally required to be made public. The same transparency spirit will be extended to the conflicts of interest declarations of trialists and those of the independent members of the oversight committees who will be required to publicly post these documents at the start and periodically update them. The involvement of the patients, carers, and the public will also be required to be described with any conflicts of interests of the citizen co-investigators declared.

Conflicts of interest: Potential or perceived compromise in the objectivity or judgment of anyone involved in research and publication due to financial or personal (non-financial) interests. Failure of declaration is considered research misconduct.

Box 5.2: Trial sample size estimation

Background:

- Sample size estimation is educated guesswork.
- Transparent sample size estimation is a necessary requirement for an ethically justifiable trial.
- The sample size is stated *a priori* in the trial's prospective registration.
- The question addressed in sample size estimation is: What is the appropriate participant number for the trial to enable the scientific evaluation of its main objective through statistical testing of the primary hypotheses concerning the effect of the proposed intervention on the primary outcome?
- Conventionally, the above idea corresponds to the completed trial's ability to calculate the point estimate of the effect of the intervention on the primary outcome with a narrow enough confidence interval to exclude the absence of an effect.
- Sample size paradox: A smaller than required sample size (unpowered trial) risks false negative findings, while a larger-than-required sample size (overpowered trial) risks false positive findings that lack clinical value.

The *a priori* sample size estimation:

- The primary outcome is determined first. The selection of the primary outcome ought to be influenced by the importance attached to the changes in health status desired given the disease or the condition targeted by the proposed trial intervention. A core outcome set on which there is consensus among patients and practitioners that they directly measure what is relevant provides a good starting point for discussion.

- After the primary outcome is selected, an educated guess has to be made about the expectations within the trial for the group comparison between the new intervention and the control, in terms of both, the magnitude of the difference between groups and the expected width of the confidence interval.
- For hypothesis testing, the probabilities of two types of statistical errors are fixed. Erroneously finding a difference in group outcomes when in truth there is none (false positive; type I or alpha error); statistical significance level, the limit of the probability of this error, is usually set at 5% or p-value 0.05. Erroneously finding a similarity in group outcomes when in truth there is a difference (false negative; type II or beta error) is usually measured as statistical power (100% − beta) set at 80% or 90%.
- Things that may sometimes be unjustifiably used to reduce the sample size requirement: setting eligibility criteria to include higher-risk participant samples; setting the statistical power too low; proposing an unrealistically large magnitude of the outcome difference between groups; selecting surrogate outcomes based on continuous data; selecting inadequate composite outcomes designed to increase event rates; etc.

Considerations during trial conduct and analysis:
- Failure to convince the estimated number of eligible participants to take part will make for a failed trial. Recruitment rates are monitored by the trial management group throughout the trial.
- Failure to convince those who consented to remain under follow-up for the primary outcome data collection also makes for a failed trial. Losses to follow-up, drop outs and withdrawals are monitored by the trial management group throughout the trial.
- Missing outcome data may introduce attrition bias (Box 2.2) and imprecision. Additionally, it may necessitate outcome data imputation for performing intention-to-treat analyses for which the methods ought to be prespecified in the statistical analysis plan (Box 5.3).
- If the expected outcome experience overall or per group is badly judged, the total numbers required may be higher or lower than the sample size originally estimated. The data monitoring committee can evaluate this blindly and give feedback to the trial steering committee about the need for trial sample size re-estimation.

The above is relevant for a trial designed with the main objective of evaluating the superiority of the new intervention over control using frequentist statistical methods; other designs may deploy different statistical approaches; Bayesian methods are not within the scope of this book. See Box 5.3 for the statistical analysis plan.
Source: DOI: 10.1136/bmj.k3750.

Following ethics committee approval, the protocol should append the approval letter containing the approval date. Additionally, following registration, the protocol frontmatter should include the trial registration details including the registration date.

Prospective trial registration

Prospective registration, the current minimum standard for trials, is insufficient for full transparency. It is, however, the right first step. Public availability of trial information can help prevent unnecessary duplication, avoiding research waste. It is estimated that the results of only around half of all the trials ever conducted have been reported. This cannot be a tolerable situation. Even if approved trials were never completed as planned, it would be helpful to know what happened. It will help prevent investment in trials that are unlikely to succeed. The obligation to report is an ethical duty for trialists as the participants who consent to participate in good faith expect that their data will be reported, not thrown away. Prospective registration, at least in theory, increases the probability that findings will be reported. In practice, this remains nothing more than an aspiration. The International Committee of Medical Journal Editors (ICMJE) had made prospective registration a requirement for publication in mid-2005. An evaluation over a decade after this directive was disappointing. It found that only around four of every 10 trials published in PubMed journals in 2018 were prospectively publicly registered (DOI: 10.1136bmj.m982). Coordinated campaigns, such as AllTrials and RIAT, aim to have all past and present trials publicly registered and correctly reported.

The key benefit of prospective registration is its ability to minimize selective outcome reporting, a questionable research practice. It is associated with publication bias, the result of a questionable publication practice where journals prioritize positive findings regardless of trial integrity and quality. The trial results reported in the published trial should be for the same outcomes as those listed in the prospective registration. The listing of results reported should be complete and ordered in importance according to the order of the outcomes prospectively registered, not determined retrospectively according to statistical significance. The originally registered primary outcome should be verified by editors and peer reviewers before publication (something they do not always do thoroughly; see Box 7.3 for a case study). Unexplained discrepancies may raise concerns over integrity. Those appraising trials may have questions and trialists should address all enquiries made. The transparency afforded by prospective registration helps trialists demonstrate their commitment to the open science.

The ICMJE, which helps self-regulate healthcare journals, had advised that all trials starting recruitment from mid-2005 onwards should be prospectively registered, i.e., registration should occur before the first participant is enrolled. It required the putting in practice, i.e., the enforcement, of this policy as a condition for publication of trials by its member journals. If a delay occurs between the submission by the trialists and the

AllTrials: A campaign for all past and present clinical trials to be registered and their methods and summary results reported (alltrials.net).

RIAT: An international effort to restoring invisible (unpublished) and abandoned (misreported) trials (restoringtrials.org).

Selective outcome reporting: A difference in the outcomes in a published trial compared to its ethics committee-approved protocol. Prospective registration encourages reporting the result for the original primary outcome, even if it shows a statistically non-significant result on trial completion.

Journal: An establishment composed of editors and other publishing staff who organize peer reviews of trial manuscripts and their publication.

uploading of the registration by the registry due to technical reasons, then this is not the trialists' fault. Trialists should record their submission to the registry with date and time stamps. Note that date and time stamps are geographically bound. As the time zones may differ across countries, trialists should be mindful of this issue. Journals ought to be sensible when applying these ICMJE policies. How to define first participant enrolment? The date and time of the first participant's consent is recommended. Trialists should note that the consent forms should record both, the date and time, where relevant.

Defining publicly accessible registration is made easy by linkage to the World Health Organization (WHO) International Clinical Trials Registry Platform which provides the minimum data items for registration. The approval of a trial by a human research ethics committee is not considered equivalent to or a substitute for the prospective registration requirement by journals. As part of its approval, human research ethics committees should make prospective registration an obligation for trialists before approaching potential participants for consent. Trialists are expected to include the registration details in the published papers and to update their registries with details of journal citations on publication of trial outputs such as protocols, conference abstracts or posters, and papers with trial results.

Given the importance of trials for healthcare, the AllTrials campaign rightly wants all past and present trials to be registered and publicly reported. Therefore, a trial not prospectively registered would have to be retrospectively registered. The ICMJE enforcement of its prospective registration rule as a condition for publication by its member journals creates a little difficulty here. However, there is flexibility in some journals, for example, PLoS One, that permit publication of trial results with retrospective registration as long as an explanation for the failure to prospectively register is provided and the implications discussed.

Statistical analysis plan

It is well known that journals tend to prioritize statistically significant results for publication. Cherry picking, fishing expeditions, harking, and p-hacking, are all forms of manipulation of data analysis to produce statistically significant results (see Glossary). These issues are linked to selective outcome reporting, a problem addressed by prospective trial registration. However, this alone is not sufficient protection. Even when it is not possible to manipulate the trial outcomes, it is possible to manipulate statistical methods in the analysis of the primary outcome in a sophisticated form of p-hacking. To avoid this problem a key requirement is that the trial dataset is not given for analysis to the trial statistician until a detailed statistical analysis plan has been specified.

International Committee of Medical Journal Editors (ICMJE): Guidance to journals on publishing policies such as public registration of clinical trials (icmje.org).

Institution: A clinical academic organization, such as a university or a hospital, where trials take place. Institutions have primary responsibility for the ethical and professional conduct of their trials.

The statistical analysis provided in the approved protocol tends to be in outline form (Box 5.2). While this may be sufficient for assessment by the peer reviewers of funding bodies and human research ethics committees, it should specify the primary analysis, such as the statistical methods to be applied to test the hypothesis concerning the intervention effect on the primary outcome. However, it may have room for maneuver. Depending on the trial design and timeframe, and the level of detail given in the approved protocol, the analysis plan initially drafted may be sufficient. The decision about whether a more detailed statistical analysis plan will be required ought to be formally made at the start and documented in the protocol. Perhaps the funder or the ethics committee will make this a condition in their approval. The timing of the preparation of the statistical analysis plan may also be dictated by the requirements placed by drug and device regulators.

During the course of the trial, toward the end of the recruitment period and before the database closure, a more complete analysis plan should be formally prepared giving the technical details of the statistical methods to be deployed and their justification (Box 5.3). This should happen without the knowledge of the outcome data. The maintenance of confidentiality during data collection and then the locking of database to prevent unauthorized changes to it after follow-up completion are key to trial integrity (Chapter 6). The date-stamped statistical analysis plan should be prospectively published publicly in unredacted form. This must happen in advance of the data becoming available to the trial statistician after the trial database is locked. Trialists should go over and above the current minimum transparency standards to regain trust. There is currently no technological barrier to achieving this.

The approved protocol should be sufficiently detailed to guide data collection. The trial protocol should contain the case report forms. Once collected, the data will be entered into the trial database. The trialists are kept blind to the outcome data. The detailed formal statistical analysis plan should specify exactly how the hypotheses associated with the objectives will be tested. It should contain a comprehensive set of instructions, which should be replicable by independent third parties such as the statisticians deployed by journals reviewing the submitted manuscript. For the primary analysis outlined in the protocol, a single analysis strategy should be specified. Any additional analyses to be undertaken should be earmarked as supplementary. For example, an intention-to-treat analysis, undertaken according to participants' initial group allocation, independent of whether they dropped out, requires an outcome (whether observed or estimated) for all participants. For such an analysis, there are many ways to deal with dropouts. One method should be specified as the primary analysis and the others as sensitivity analysis. Whether the baseline characteristics and the stratification or minimization variable used in

Cherry-picking: Reporting particular data and results while omitting others, a practice associated with the performance of multiple statistical tests in a dataset (fishing expedition) until one of them turns up significant, for example, the p-value observed crosses the statistical significance threshold (p-hacking).

Regulator: A formal body set up for official approvals of medicines and devices, for example, the European Medicines Agency (EMA), and the US Food and Drug Administration (FDA).

random sequence generation will be included as covariates in a primary statistical analysis or not should be specified.

Not all the information required for the analysis plan is available at the time of writing the protocol. Assumptions are made about many factors, for example, sample size is inflated considering the possibility of dropout. For some assumptions, data becomes available during the course of the trial, such as adherence to the intervention, dropout rates, and more. The data monitoring committee may permit the sharing of this type of information with the trialists (without unblinding the outcome data). Such information can help in preparing the statistical analysis plan. For example, if it is known that the dropout rate is extremely low, a complete case analysis may be most expedient as the primary analytic strategy (excluding the small proportion of participants with missing outcome data). Even if such information is not shared with trialists, some objective decision rules can be set *a priori* to direct the analytic strategy. For example, the dropout rate below which complete case analysis will be deployed as the primary analysis can be pre-specified. The idea behind this approach is to reduce the room for maneuver in the data analysis to the minimum. Some other fixes may be used to maximize statistical power in the final analysis. For example, comparison with baseline to measure change in continuous outcome data, and making adjustments in multivariable models for baseline characteristics and the stratification or minimization variables deployed in random sequence generation. Unless pre-specified in the statistical analysis plan, they are tantamount to p-hacking.

Sensitivity analysis: Repetition of an analysis under different assumptions to examine the impact of these assumptions on the result.

Intention-to-treat: An analysis where participants are analyzed according to their initial group allocation, independent of whether they dropped out, fully complied with the intervention, or not. A true intention-to-treat analysis includes an outcome (whether observed or estimated) for all participants randomized.

Box 5.3: Suggested trial statistical analysis plan outline

Title page and front matter:
- Trial name, registrations and protocol details, names, and institutions of the trialists.
- Names and institutions of the statistical analysis plan authors.
- Version number and date (necessary to easily recognize modifications).

Background:
- Objectives and related hypotheses (specify the main objective and its related primary hypothesis).
- The sample size estimation in the protocol and relevant assumptions (revisit statistical considerations in the protocol as the statistical analysis plan must correspond with it).
- Prospectively registered outcomes, both primary and secondary (specify in terms of measurements).

Statistical analyses:

- The primary analysis: Test the primary hypothesis related to the main objective focusing on the primary outcome measure using a single pre-specified analytic strategy (key analytic considerations include intention-to-treat analysis, handling of missing outcome data, adjustment of the analysis for baseline characteristics and the variables used in stratification or minimization deployed in random sequence generation, statistical methods, and tests, pre-specification of significance level if there are multiple primary outcomes or p-value adjustment for multiple statistical testing, etc.).
- The secondary analyses: Cover any additional analyses of the primary outcome (complete case analysis, per protocol analysis, subgroup analysis, and sensitivity analysis) and the analyses of the secondary outcomes.
- Exploratory data analyses.

The above is not a complete list; templates vary depending on requirements. Data monitoring and confidential interim analyses require their own statistical planning (Chapter 6). The statistical analysis plan should be prospectively published publicly before locking the trial database after the completion of the follow-up of the last randomized participant.
See Box 5.2 for sample size estimation.
See Box 3.1 for grey areas in responsible research conduct, e.g., even for the prospectively registered primary outcome the door to the possibility of p-hacking remains open through the multiple options available for the primary analysis; pre-specification of a single analytic strategy offers a transparent solution.
Source: DOI: 10.1186/s12916-020-01706-7.

The pre-specified statistical analysis plan will be implemented using statistical software. The codes and outputs from these analyses will form the basis of the results to be reported. These codes and outputs should be shared transparently along with the manuscript of the trial paper. Any modifications made to the statistical analysis plan must be provided in the trial manuscript with justification. If the statistical analysis plan is prepared early in the course of the trial, there remains the possibility that the trial protocol may need to be modified, e.g., trial sample size may be changed in light of the more detailed consideration. Any such modification should be reported in the method section of the trial manuscript and the implications should be discussed to maximize transparency (Chapter 7).

Chapter 5: Trial planning – Key points

Execution of trials (advice to trialists)

- Ensure patient, carer, and public involvement in determining trial priority, participant eligibility, intervention feasibility, outcome importance, trial acceptability, consent form development, and patient information pack preparation.
- Register the trial on a recognized registry before the first participant is approached for consent.
- Publish the human research ethics committee approved trial protocol, consent form, and patient information (Chapter 4). Ideally, publish the protocol in a peer-reviewed journal.
- Publicly post conflicts of interest declarations of all trialists, citizens involved in trial co-production, and independent members of trial oversight committees (Chapter 6), and periodically update them. Publish these in the protocol and the final paper containing trial results.
- Prepare the statistical analysis plan before the dataset is locked for analysis. Publish the *a priori* statistical analysis plan on the online prospective registration or another open science platform. Include preparation of the statistical analysis plan as one of the roles when detailing contributions in the trial's authorship (Box 8.2).
- Follow the approved protocol. Any deviations, whether planned and unplanned, should be reported with results honestly in the manuscript prepared for submission.
- After trial completion, post the main results on the registry (ideally within 12 months). Keep this brief as a precaution in case a journal reprimands trialists for having a prior publication when considering the main manuscript. However, the world has moved on. Nowadays, preprints are not considered disqualifiers for submission. Journals actively offer posting of the submitted manuscript on their preprint partner servers. Trialists should take up this option without hesitation to maximize transparency.
- Include registration details in the publication of all trial outputs such as protocol, statistical analysis plan, conference abstracts or posters, preprints, and papers with trial results.

Writing tips for trial authors

- See related key points in Chapters 6 and 7.
- **Title:** Give registration details following the journal's authors'

Research priority: The ranking or selection of a few among the many established research gaps and needs.

Research gap: A gap in knowledge.

Research need: A research gap resulting in an inability to make healthcare decisions.

Preprint: A publicly posted draft version of a manuscript, usually simultaneously posted at the first submission to a journal, and is available prior to completion of its formal peer review. Preprints usually have DOIs (digital object identifiers) and can be cited like any other paper.

Contributor Roles Taxonomy (CRediT): A system for classifying the roles played by individual authors and those acknowledged in a trial publication.

instructions. The unique trial registration number should be provided.

- **Abstract:** Provide registration details. Focus on the findings related to the primary outcome.
- **Methods:** Give the ethics committee approval date, registration date, and the date of consent of the first participant. Describe the intervention trialed in sufficient detail to permit replication in future trials and practice. State if any deviations from approved protocol, planned and unplanned, took place in the course of the trial. Provide information about any modifications to the intervention outlined in the protocol. Provide information about adherence to the intervention. Justify sample size estimation based on the primary outcome registered in a manner that permits replication by others. Give dates of the statistical analysis plan, completion of follow-up of the last participant, and locking of the dataset after data entry closure. Provide details of where the statistical analysis plan can be found and give the corresponding analysis codes and output as supplementary material. Give data sharing details.
- **Results:** Give the number of participants lost at each stage of the trial and the number of participants with data loss explicitly (best done via a flow diagram). Strictly stick to the primary outcome originally registered.
- **Tables and figures:** In the tabulation of results the outcomes should be listed in the same order as that originally registered (do not reorder according to statistical significance). Report explicitly and completely in a way that allows replication of statistical tests based on reported data without the need to access raw data as much as possible.
- **Discussion:** Avoid spin altogether. Give the implications of any modifications to the originally approved protocol as part of the trial's strengths and limitations. Ensure that the trial conclusion is bound within any limitations placed by the modifications.
- **Funding disclosures:** Given full account of direct funding to the trial.
- **Supplementary material:** Provide the date-stamped human research ethics committee approval documentation. Provide date-stamped trial protocol and consent form with accompanying patient information (Chapter 4). Provide the date-stamped *a priori* statistical analysis plan if not already linked in the methods section. Share the statistical analysis codes and outputs to back the results presented.

Roles of institutions, funders, and journals

- Funders should make prospective registration including data sharing plans a condition for funding trials.
- Human research ethics committees should make prospective registration including data sharing plans a condition to be met after approval.
- Institutions, funders, and journals should seek prospective publication of trial protocols and statistical analysis plans.

6 *Trial oversight*

Trialist: An investigator who contributes to a trial and is credited in the authorship or the acknowledgment section of the published article.

Once approved and prospectively registered, trials benefit from independent oversight provided by trial steering and data monitoring committees. Participant safety in terms of their healthcare and safeguarding their rights and well-being take priority over any scientific objectives in this phase of the trial; the trial may be modified or stopped at any stage to protect participants. The independent input is additional to the institutional research governance arrangements for supervising research. Prospective and continuous public documentation of trials throughout their lifecycle is going to go further than the current transparency requirement for trial registration with data sharing plans. As things develop in the open science arena, there is a real possibility that all non-confidential parts of reports of governance audits, inspections, and the formal minutes and papers of trial steering and independent data monitoring committees will be expected to be made public contemporaneously. The conflicts of interest declarations of the independent members of the trial oversight committees should be publicly posted at the start and periodically updated. This chapter will guide trialists on how to ensure compliance with professional standards in the conduct of approved trials.

Institution: A clinical academic organization, for example, a university or a hospital, where trials take place.

Research governance: The system set up by institutions to oversee that the conduct of trials under their auspices are in compliance with regulations.

An outline of trial management

Trial management group: Group comprising of co-investigators and appointed trial staff, led by the chief investigator to oversee the conduct of the trial.

Once approved by the human research ethics committee, the trial can proceed. It must obtain approval from the research governance office of each institution that will serve as a site for participant enrolment and follow-up. Without consenting, eligible participants, there cannot be a trial. Likewise, without outcome data, a trial cannot exist. The pursuit of enrolling participants, randomizing them to the groups allocated, and following them to obtain their outcome data is what one might describe as trial conduct.

Designing the trial protocol, obtaining ethics committee approval, and prospective registration precede trial conduct. The trial conduct commences with the consenting of the first participant and ends with data analysis according to the *a priori* statistical analysis plan undertaken after the last participant has completed follow-up. Throughout this time, the participant's safety and the protection of their rights and well-being must remain the top priority. The chief investigator should establish a trial management group, that will deliver the trial under the oversight of institutional research governance. Trials may be subjected to audits and inspections. During the course of the trial, depending on trial design, complexity, and regulations, trialists might benefit from external, independent input. If assessed as a condition or requirement, the setting

DOI: 10.1201/9781003461401-6

up of trial steering and independent data monitoring committees may be mandated by human research ethics committees, funders, or regulators (see below). This supervision will help to instill and ensure research integrity during this part of the trial's lifecycle.

Research governance

Institutions where trials take place, are legally required to set up research governance offices to oversee the conduct of research undertaken within their umbrella. Trialists, including chief investigators, site principal investigators, clinical investigators, and others can engage in trials only with their approval and remain under their oversight throughout the trial. The institutional research governance approval is additional to the human research ethics committee approval (Chapter 4).

The research governance office ensures the compliance of approved trials with ethical and professional standards for the conduct of human clinical research. This standard, known as Good Clinical Practice in human clinical trials or GCP, is widely used and applied across the entire lifecycle of the trial, including documentation of informed consent, participant safety monitoring, data integrity, and more. The name GCP itself is a misnomer as the standard pertains to research in humans in the form of clinical trials, not to clinical practice. GCP primarily targets trials undertaken to obtain regulatory approval. However, most trials are not undertaken for this purpose. There is no reason why non-regulatory trials should be undertaken to meet a lower standard. Concerns have been raised that GCP is a cumbersome standard. All standards should be reviewed and updated periodically. Trialists should work towards making their best effort over and above what is required as the minimum standard.

Research governance offices undertake audits and are subjected to inspections for their oversight of trials. They have a program of audits to examine and address possible integrity risks early on. To conduct a trial with fidelity to its approved protocol and professional standards is a dynamic process. Research governance includes an evaluation of the trial's compliance with its approved protocol and with professional standards such as the GCP. This audit may include an examination of trial activities (e.g., informed consent), and documents (e.g., data collection and recording). This is a part of what is known as "quality assurance" and is usually undertaken as a planned formal activity. It aims to assist trialists in meeting professional standards, preparing for external audits, and demonstrating robust research processes to external bodies including

Chief investigator: The trialist, in some academic cultures also known as the principal investigator, responsible for the conduct of the whole trial throughout its lifecycle from inception to publication. The chief investigator heads the trial management group.

Audit: A planned formal evaluation of trial conduct, i.e., activities (e.g., informed consent), and documents (e.g., data collection and recording), to independently determine if the trial is compliant with its approved protocol and meets professional standards such as Good Clinical Practice in human clinical trials (GCP).

Inspection: An audit conducted by an external legally competent authority, that has serious implications for the trialists and their institutions in case of a finding of non-compliance with professional standards such as Good Clinical Practice in human clinical trials (GCP).

funders and journals. Audits are meant to protect trial participants and they assist institutions in identifying and meeting the training needs of trialists they employ.

An inspection is, in simple terms, an audit conducted by an external legally competent authority. It has serious implications for the trialists and their institution in case of non-compliance. It goes without saying that all trial-related activities and documentation should be continuously maintained in a state of readiness for audits and inspections. In cases of funded trials and trials conducted for regulatory approval, the sword of external audits and inspections will always be hanging over the trialists' heads. The details of such inspections are outside the scope of this book. Instead of fear of reprimand, ensuring participant protection and trial integrity should be the motive here for trialists. The reports of audits and inspections that have taken place may also be shared at the time of publication to reassure editors, peer reviewers, and readers about trial trustworthiness.

Sponsor: Clinical trial regulations require that a sponsor makes proper arrangements to initiate and conduct trials. For trialists employed in an academic setting, it is usually their own institution that acts as the sponsor.

Funder: Organizations such as governmental agencies, philanthropists, research charities, and industries that provide funding for a trial under contract to an institution.

Box 6.1: A trial's oversight and management structure

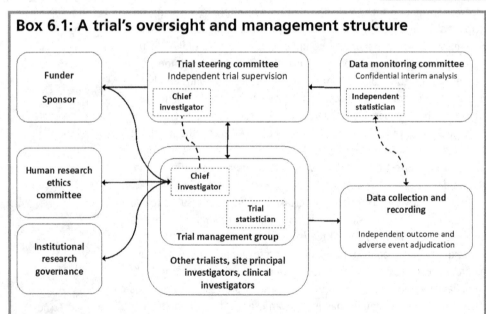

Structures may vary across jurisdictions and from trial to trial.
Dashed lines with arrows: confidential data access and analysis during the trial's course; outcome data by group is not accessed by trialists until the last randomized participant has completed follow-up, the a priori statistical analysis plan has been published (Box 5.3) and the database has been locked.

Trial management group

The trial management group led by the chief investigator is responsible for the day-to-day conduct of the trial to achieve the sample size required with complete participant follow-up within the agreed timeframe (Box 6.1). Depending on the trial size and available funding, the trialist team would include a trial manager and trial coordinators in addition to site principal investigators and clinical investigators. The trial management group will ensure that all trial investigators follow the ethics committee-approved trial protocol. The protocol is a live document. It would have to be initially agreed with the trial steering and independent data monitoring committees and then reviewed regularly. There may be changes to the protocol from time to time, and the ethics committee would need to be kept informed and reapproval obtained in case of substantial amendments. Participant safety monitoring and adverse event reporting is a key task during the trial. The trialist team members may have some training requirements, for example, GCP certification and consent training. There will be the need to prepare a delegation log to ensure that all trialists have their roles and responsibilities clarified to them. The trial team will need to engage with research governance. Communication is a key challenge in trials with many investigators involved. The trial management group will need to report to the trial steering committee and implement the advice received as part of independent supervision, if required.

Site principal investigator: The trialist or investigator coordinating all trial affairs in a trial site or center. There can be no trial without randomized participants who have complete follow-up data. So, this role is recognized in trial authorship or acknowledgment.

Clinical investigator: Healthcare professionals who execute trials in clinical practice according to the approved protocol, including signing up trial participants and obtaining their informed consent.

Data collection and recording

The case report from, a paper-based or an electronic document, is the tool that collects the data from consented, eligible participants. This is the source data. This data is entered into the trial master database and will be used for statistical analysis and reporting. The trial, during its course, has the raw data accumulating, i.e., the data being collected on the case report from every participant is continuously recorded in the master database electronically. From this, after data cleaning and possibly some restructuring, an analysis file will be extracted after the raw database is locked upon completion of the follow-up of the last randomized participant. The data analysis specified in the *a priori* statistical analysis plan will be applied to this dataset. This is also the dataset which will be shared publicly in deidentified or anonymized form on trial completion.

Database development and management is a science in its own right. Institutions are required to provide training to trialists and establish a secure infrastructure for this. Trial data integrity is an integral part of research integrity. Data entry should be attributable and individuals who enter data and make changes to it should be identifiable. The database

Case report form: A paper-based or electronic document used for data collection from each consenting participant in a trial. Once collected, the data is entered into the trial database used for statistical analysis and reporting.

passwords and access criteria are therefore all important in trial management. All modifications to data should be traceable. Mechanisms should be put in place to avoid unauthorized modifications. The data should be recorded contemporaneously so that errors identified through automated checks can be rectified before it is too late. The original case report forms should always be kept securely so it is possible to get back to the source data. All variable coding should be complete to permit independent data analysis, i.e., there is a need to create metadata to accompany the shared data. The protection of participant confidentiality and privacy are key issues in data collection and recording (and data sharing following trial completion), as any breaches could risk legal consequences for the institutions involved in the trial. Needless to say, trialists have to act responsibly in this regard with the support of their institutions.

During the course of the trial, the accumulating trial data should be available for confidential interim analysis by the independent data monitoring committee, if required. The interim analysis plan should be pre-specified and incorporated into the trial protocol. The outcome data per group should never be available to trialists, until after the *a priori* statistical analysis plan has been published and the trial database has been locked after the completion of the follow-up of the last randomized participant. In case of subjective outcomes and adverse events, trialists may establish an outcome adjudication committee, ideally made up of independent experts who are kept blind to participants' group allocation. This approach aims to standardize outcome assessment against protocol-specified criteria, minimizing the risk of measurement bias in trials with subjectivity in these assessments. Adverse events classification may also benefit from independent adjudication to determine whether they are serious or not and related to intervention or not. See the case study concerning trial restoration following independent outcome re-adjudication in Box 2.6.

Assessing the need for independent oversight

Trials come in all shapes and sizes, each very different from the other (Box 1.2). The independent oversight arrangements described above are typically recommended for those trials that come all singing, all dancing, i.e., full of promise of clinical usefulness (Box 2.5). Trials undertaken for regulatory approval have to set up oversight arrangements as dictated by the regulators. Funders may also place particular requirements for oversight of the trials they fund. Outside the regulatory environment, the oversight arrangements should be proportional to trial complexity. Trialists would have made their assessment of the risk as part of their application for the human research ethics committee approval (Chapter 4).

Outcome adjudication committee: Outcomes, including adverse events, may be best adjudicated by independent experts or trialists blind to participants' group allocation who standardize outcome assessment against protocol-specified criteria, minimizing the risk of measurement bias.

Adverse event: An undesirable and unintended harmful or unpleasant occurrence associated with an intervention. If there is a suggestion of a causal relationship, the term used is "adverse reaction".

Regulator: A formal body set up for official approvals of medicines and devices, such as the European Medicines Agency (EMA), the US Food and Drug Administration (FDA), and the UK Medicines and Healthcare products Regulatory Agency (MHRA).

There is an obligation to meet the fundamental research ethics principle of non-maleficence (do no harm). The ethics committee should give guidance on the intensity of oversight for participant protection if it assesses the risk to be different than that judged by trialists.

The complexity of a trial depends on many factors, with size being one key feature. A trial with a large sample size may be expected to recruit over several years, and the risk to participants may change over time. Note that explanatory or pilot trials may not be regarded as simple just because they are small in size. The level of risk to participants, intervention-related and disease-related, are both key. The participants may be vulnerable, without the capacity to consent, or at risk of suffering poor outcomes. This risk may be due to the type of group allocation, for example, the risk under no treatment or placebo may be higher than that under standard healthcare. In the control group, participants' safety has to be prioritized as much as in the intervention group. The intervention itself may be complex or invasive. Adverse event monitoring thus becomes a key issue as affected participants may require specific treatment. Depending on the seriousness of the issue, alteration of the intervention may also be required to protect future participants and the protocol modification would need to pass through ethics committee re-approval. If the participants' safety is compromised, the trial will be required to be stopped early, guided by the formal assessment of the independent data monitoring committee.

Their trial and its participants stand to benefit from independent oversight if the trialist team is inexperienced. Many countries do not have well-prepared medical infrastructure and little to no experience in conducting trials. If an agreement can be reached that a trial can be defined as low risk, it may not need independent oversight. The oversight provided by the research governance office of the institution may suffice in this case. If there is any doubt about the level of risk being sufficiently low, the independent trial supervision model outlined in the trial management structure above should be followed (Box 6.1). The bottom line is that all trials need oversight to protect participants during their conduct, regardless of the level of trial complexity. The question of intensity of the oversight should be addressed proportionate to the assessed level of risk to the trial participants. Where indicated by the level of trial complexity and risk, independent oversight should be used as extra protection over and above the mandatory institutional research governance office oversight.

Non-maleficence:
The fundamental research ethics principle that potential risks to trial participants should be balanced against the benefits gained from undertaking trials.

Trial steering committee

Not all trials will be formally required to have a trial steering committee with an independent chair, but to safeguard trial integrity, there is no reason why as part of responsible research practice trialists should not spontaneously establish one. The steering committee is responsible for the overall supervision of the trial. The steering committee consists of an independent chair, independent members including patient representatives, the chief investigator, and other senior trialists from the trial management group. The committee membership should have relevant scientific, healthcare, and clinical trial experience. In multi-country trials involving less developed settings, the membership should be international, including independent experts who have experience in trials in such settings. The independent chair should not be an employee of the trialist's institution and should not be involved in the trial in any way other than in the steering committee role. The declarations of the conflicts of interest of the independent members of the steering committee should be publicly posted at the start and periodically updated. The members of the independent steering committee are not named as authors in the published trial outputs; they are acknowledged (Chapter 8). For this reason, sometimes trialists might find it difficult to recruit experienced independent colleagues for the steering committee as such individuals tend to be busy and prioritize their own research work.

The steering committee advises the trial management group, the sponsor, and the funder. Its role covers, among other things, ensuring research integrity of the trial by meeting ethical and professional standards. At its first meeting, which may be held jointly with the data monitoring committee, the independent members should provide feedback to trialists on the protocol, the informed consent, and the patient information. Assessing adherence to the approved trial protocol and the statistical analysis plan is a key committee role. Assessing trial progress against the timeline agreed is essential for delivering the trial as planned. Participant safety assessment is one of the most important roles of the steering committee. Depending on the confidential evaluation of the evidence accumulating in the trial by the data monitoring committee, the steering committee should provide advice to trialists regarding continuing, modifying, or terminating the trial. This advice would also depend on any new external information, such as the publication of the results of other trials, that may emerge during the course of the trial. Trialists should keep the systematic reviews they undertook at the time of protocol preparation updated throughout the course of the trial (Chapter 9). The modifications may involve changes to the protocol, the patient information for obtaining informed consent, and more. Any modifications should be presented to the ethics committee. Finally, on trial completion, the steering committee should ensure timely dissemination of the trial's findings. Apart from providing a report of the main findings to the ethics committee and updating the trial registry with these findings, trialists should publish in a journal. The steering committee role should advise on meeting the transparency requirements for publication including responsible data sharing

Citizen science: An open science initiative encouraging public and consumer involvement in scientific research, with citizens actively making intellectual contributions.

Systematic review: A method of summarizing the evidence using systematic and explicit methods to identify, select, and appraise relevant primary studies, and to extract, collate, and report their findings.

Meta-analysis: A statistical technique for combining (pooling) the results of multiple trials addressing the same question to produce a summary result.

Journal: An establishment composed of editors and other publishing staff who organize peer reviews of trial manuscripts and their publication.

(Chapter 7). Some regulatory trials may have restrictions placed on them, but otherwise data sharing should be the norm. The steering committee, as part of its role in dissemination, should also direct trialists to update and publish systematic reviews with meta-analysis including the trial's findings (Chapter 9).

In large trials that run over the course of several years and do not present a high risk to participants, the steering committee might meet annually. The chief investigator may request additional meetings, if required, to assess and advise on any urgent issues. All steering committee records have to be kept safe by the trialist team. These records may have to be made available on request, in case integrity concerns are raised. To protect against such complaints, the steering committee should obtain a certificate of data integrity from the data monitoring committee and present it as part of the submission of the trial manuscript to a journal (Box 7.6). The most transparent approach would be for the steering committee minutes and papers to be made public contemporaneously.

Independent data monitoring committee

The data monitoring committee is made up of a group of independent experts who confidentially review the accumulating trial data on a regular basis in order to examine the continuing safety of the participants during the course of the trial. It is also sometimes called the "data and safety monitoring board". The data monitoring committee membership should be completely independent of the trial. The conflicts of interest declarations of the monitoring committee members should be publicly posted at the start and periodically updated. The data monitoring committee members are not named as authors in the published trial outputs; they are acknowledged (Chapter 8).

The independent data monitoring committee has access to the accumulating trial data (including outcome data by group allocation if required). Note that trialists are not given access to trial data during the course of the trial, as they only access the database after it has been locked following the collection of the outcome data from the last randomized participant and the statistical analysis plan has been finalised. The data monitoring committee advises the trial steering committee, which in turn communicates with the chief investigator, sponsor, and funder through its independent chair. It recommends whether to continue the trial as planned, modify its protocol, or stop the trial early. For making this recommendation, it may decide to undertake confidential interim analyses of accumulating trial data. The results of interim analyses are not shared with the trialists. If it evaluates the adverse events recorded in the trial as being serious, the participant recruitment may be

Data Monitoring Committee (DMC), composed of independent experts, reports to the Trial Steering Committee (TSC), making recommendations regarding trial continuation, modification, or termination. TSC, composed of an independent chair and members as well as some of the trialists, is responsible for overall trial supervision, and its chair gives instructions to the trial management group.

paused to evaluate safety. Any confidential interim analyses and rules for stopping the trial early should be pre-specified, and the protocol updated with the interim statistical analysis plan. The details of statistical issues in confidential interim analysis are outside the scope of this book, but in simple terms, the following possibilities may transpire. If these analyses determine that the trial intervention is harmful against pre-specified criteria, the monitoring committee can recommend stopping the trial early to protect the intervention group. It may also be able to find the trial intervention effective under some circumstances, and can recommend stopping the trial early to protect the control group from continuing exposure in the trial to inferior healthcare (Box 2.6). When making these assessments, in addition to the accumulating trial data, the monitoring committee should also consider the findings of any ongoing trials published. Conducting an interim analysis often has implications for the statistical analysis plan of the completed trial (Box 5.3). Therefore, the data monitoring committee should have the opportunity to comment on the statistical analysis plan and the manuscript of the trial's findings before submission. The data monitoring committee should also give a certificate of data integrity to accompany the publication of the trial findings (Box 7.6).

The data monitoring committee should meet in time to provide its report to the trial steering committee's scheduled meetings. The content of the data monitoring report should be agreed upon at its first committee meeting. The need for confidential interim analyses, their timings, and stopping rules should be pre-specified early, and incorporated into the trial protocol. The report for the data monitoring committee should be prepared sufficiently in advance to a proper evaluation. The report usually has two parts, an open part on data about trial progress, and a part on the confidential interim analysis. Although the trial statistician can be involved in preparing these reports, they will unnecessarily have to take the burden of responsibility for maintaining confidentiality. Therefore, an independent statistician should ideally undertake this task. The data monitoring committee meetings consist of open and closed sessions; the latter is where only independent committee members meet. Open sessions may include the chief investigator, other trialists, and a trial statistician. Depending on the seriousness of the independent data monitoring committee recommendation, members of the trial steering committee, and representatives of the sponsor or funder may also be invited to attend. No trialist or trial steering committee member should attend the closed session, where trial data is evaluated. The meeting notes of open and closed sessions should be kept separate. All data monitoring committee records have to be kept safe. It is important to ensure that the confidential parts of the independent data monitoring committee deliberations and results of interim analyses are not shared during the

Statistical analysis plan: The development of the analysis outlined in a trial registration and protocol into a detailed *a priori* statistical analysis plan of the primary outcome, the secondary outcomes, and other variables before the dataset is locked and prepared for formal analysis.

Box 6.2: A proposal for a trial's complete and contemporaneous public documentation during its lifecycle

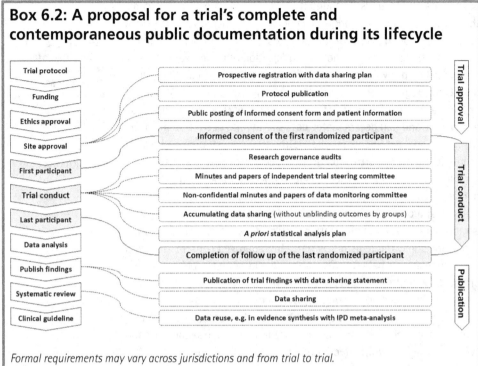

Formal requirements may vary across jurisdictions and from trial to trial.
Trial conduct commences with the consenting of the first participant and ends with data analysis according to the a priori statistical analysis plan undertaken after the last participant has completed follow-up.
See Box 3.3 for an open science vision for randomized clinical trials.
See Box 7.6 for the specification of instructions to authors for journals to publish trials responsibly.
See Box 9.1 for the role of evidence synthesis alongside trials.
See Box 9.2 for understanding evidence synthesis terminology; IPD abbreviation for individual participant data.

---

trial. These may have to be made available on request by trial completion. The non-confidential part of the data monitoring committee minutes, papers, and their recommendation made for the trial should be contemporaneously made public for transparency.

Towards more complete and contemporaneous public documentation

There is no doubt that healthcare research will move in this direction inevitably as the openness agenda will expand across all life spheres from politics to business to science. Prospective and continuous public documentation of trials throughout their lifecycle is going to become the norm (Box 6.2). There are no technological barriers to this expected development. Online platforms already exist to make this a reality today, should the trialists and stakeholder organizations choose to adopt them.

The first step toward public documentation was taken in 2005, when prospective registration was mandated by the International Committee of Medical Journal Editors (ICMJE). This is now part of the distant past. Around one and half decades later, data sharing has been recommended, with plans and statements required in the trial's registration and manuscripts (Chapter 7). Further progress is needed to take place for more complete and contemporaneous public documentation. Following the human research ethics committee approval, the protocol with the date-stamped approval letter appended should be made public. Following registration, the protocol front matter should include the trial registration details including the registration date. The approved consent form and the accompanying patient information should be made public. Further protocol, consent forms, and patient information versions should also be provided publicly whenever they are updated.

The trialists and the independent oversight committee members should make declarations of conflicts of interest public at the start and keep them regularly updated throughout the trial. There is no reason why some of the ongoing trial data, such as the total number of participants accumulating over time and their basic demographic characteristics, cannot be responsibly shared as participants are enrolled during the course of the trial. These data are already shared internally with the trial management group, the steering committee, and the data monitoring committee (in its open session) as part of trial oversight. Sharing it publicly will not do any harm and will maximize transparency. This initiative will require careful attention to protecting participant confidentiality and privacy in the same way as it is required throughout the trial. It will also need to ensure the maintenance of blinding of the trialists to outcome data by group allocation (only the independent data monitoring committee should have access to this data during the course of the trial). Moving forward, all non-confidential parts of reports of research governance audits, any inspections, and the minutes and papers of trial steering and data monitoring committees will be expected to be made public contemporaneously. The *a priori* statistical analysis plan should be shared publicly before the dataset is locked (Chapter 5). Following trial completion and at the time of publication of trial findings, or as soon as feasible afterward, the raw data should be publicly shared (Chapter 7).

International Committee of Medical Journal Editors (ICMJE): Provides guidance to journals on publishing policies such as public registration of clinical trials (icmje.org).

Chapter 6: Trial oversight – Key points

Execution of trials (advice to trialists)

- Include plans for trial oversight in the trial protocol, including the justification for independent oversight in light of the assessed trial complexity and the potential risk to participants (Chapter 4).
- Work closely with the research governance office to ensure that the trial and trial staff can get the support they need to deliver the trial with research integrity. Ensure that staff training requirements are identified and met. Retain and publicly upload any GCP audit or inspection reports.
- Keep all trialists blind to outcome data concerning group comparisons until the follow-up of the last participant has been completed and the *a priori* statistical analysis plan has been published before locking the trial database.
- Prepare and agree on the terms of reference for trial steering and independent data monitoring committees, if required. Agree on the content of the report of the accumulating data to be prepared for the independent data monitoring committee, ideally done by an independent statistician. Any confidential interim analysis plans should be pre-specified and included in the protocol (as a protocol update if required). Retain all the correspondence related to the working of committees for independent supervision (the confidential elements should be retained by the independent chair). The conflicts of interest declarations of the independent members of the trial oversight committees should be publicly posted at the start and periodically updated. Publish these in the protocol and the final paper containing trial results.
- Keep evidence syntheses undertaken for preparing trial protocols updated (Chapter 9). If new external information emerges, such as the publication of new trial results, the trial may have to be modified or even stopped early with the input of the trial oversight committees.
- Seek human research ethics committee approvals for amended protocols, consent forms, and patient information (Chapter 4). Retain all versions of these documents.
- Seek guidance from the trial steering committee on data sharing at the time of publication of trial findings. The independent data monitoring committee, if established, should give a

Conflicts of interest: Potential or perceived compromise in the objectivity or judgment of anyone involved in research and publication due to financial or personal (non-financial) interests. Failure of declaration is considered research misconduct.

certificate of data integrity to accompany the publication of the trial findings.

- In addition to the prospective registration, consider continuous and complete public documentation of the trial by posting on-line the protocol, consent form, patient information, reports of GCP audits and inspections, and non-confidential minutes and papers of the trial steering and independent data monitoring committees (Box 6.2).

Writing tips for trial authors

- See related key points in Chapters 5 and 7.
- **Methods:** Provide details of or justification for not having inde-pendent trial supervision by trial steering and data monitoring committees. Include information on the need for adjusting the trial statistical analysis plan in light of any confidential inter-im analyses planned and undertaken by the independent data monitoring committee. If the trial is closed early before achiev-ing its planned sample size (Box 5.2), give a detailed explanation as to why with the decision dates. Give dates of the meetings of trial steering and independent data monitoring committees.
- **Discussion:** Give the strengths and limitations of the trial su-pervisory system deployed. Give implications of trial findings in light of these.
- **Acknowledgments:** Include names of independent members of trial steering and data monitoring committees. Independent members are not named as authors (Chapter 8).
- **Conflicts of interest:** Declare conflicts of interest (financial and personal) for the independent members of trial oversight committees.
- **Supplementary material:** Provide reports of research govern-ance audits and inspections. Include terms of reference and non-confidential parts of the minutes and papers of trial steer-ing and independent data monitoring committees. Give the certificate of data integrity provided by the independent data monitoring committee.

Roles of institutions, funders, and journals

- Institutions and funders should work closely in trial oversight.
- Human research ethics committees should give guidance about the need for independence in trial oversight on giving approv-al considering the assessed trial complexity and the potential risk to participants. Ethics committees should review major

Transparency in research: Open research practices including prospective registration, adherence to trial design, *a priori* statistical analysis plan, data sharing, and timely and complete public reporting.

amendments to protocols, consent forms, and patient information in a timely fashion; the amended versions that have minor revisions may be approved by the committee chair.
- Journals should seek information on any audits and inspections undertaken and independent trial oversight provided during the course of the trial to maximize transparency.

TOP: Guidelines for Transparency and Openness Promotion (TOP) in journal policies and practices (osf.io/ud578).

7 Publishing trials responsibly

Journals publish the results of completed trials. They may also publish trial protocols. They provide instructions to authors on their requirements and have an established, structured process for receiving manuscripts, making their assessments, and publishing accepted articles. Not all trials are created equal. Editors and peer reviewers deploy their expert knowledge to evaluate submitted manuscripts. A major concern is that they have a bias against publishing negative results regardless of trial integrity and quality, which drives questionable research practices such as selective outcome reporting and p-hacking. Their assessment system is not quite as good as it should be, as trials harboring integrity flaws slip through and subsequently need to be retracted. Responsible publication conduct requires that they make a concerted effort to detect integrity flaws before publishing trials. The journals' academic work mostly happens behind closed doors and those passing judgments enjoy anonymity. This secrecy needs to end as open science and transparency demand as much from journals as they do from trialists. This chapter will give guidance to trialists, editors, and peer reviewers on how to undertake trial publications responsibly.

Untrustworthy trials

Regarding trials published with integrity flaws, what is the burden of this disease? In July 2023 the Nature journal announced that "Medicine is plagued by untrustworthy clinical trials". It also suggested that a third to a quarter of published trials were faked (DOI: 10.1038/d41586-023-02299-w). Accordingly, as around 25,000–30,000 randomized clinical trials are published annually in PubMed (Box 2.3), there must be a lot of trials with integrity flaws around in the literature. What happened to the promise of publishing trials responsibly?

When media interest brings to attention a story of scientific fraud this merely represents a case report or a case series. For example, the recent Stanford and Harvard research misconduct scandals are such case reports (DOI's: 10.1038/d41586-024-00009-8; 10.1126/science.adj9568). It would not be a bad metaphor to say that this represents the tip of the iceberg, and does not capture the rate quantifiably. When the Nature journal article suggested that a third to a quarter of trials are faked, it was giving the subjective probability, a hunch or a guesstimate, of the experts it interviewed. A correspondence in the journal about this article stated that it was "not backed by independently verified data". Estimating the proportion of untrustworthy trials is challenging. This calculation

DOI: 10.1201/9781003461401-7

requires the number of trials found to have integrity flaws (numerator) divided by the total number of published trials (denominator). It would seem that performing this calculation is simple arithmetic. It is not, as outlined in the case study in Box 7.1!

The calculated proportion of untrustworthy COVID-19 trials is dramatically lower than the Nature journal guesstimate. There is a need for the proper application of prevalence research methodology in accurately estimating the proportion of trials with integrity flaws. This is going to be an intellectual challenge, as defining and determining the numerator and denominator is far from a simple task. No matter how common fake trials are, in robust research, there is no debate that trials with integrity flaws should never enter into public circulation. In research and publication practice, integrity flaws in trials should be nipped in the bud at the institutions that approve them and oversee their conduct. Moreover, integrity flaws in completed trials should be picked up by the journals assessing the trial manuscripts, preventing their publication. The Nature journal is not the only one highlighting the failures in publishing trials responsibly.

PubMed: A freely available interface of the general biomedical research database Medline, which contains citations with and without abstracts (ncbi.nlm.nih.gov/PubMed).

Box 7.1: Case study – Calculating the proportion of untrustworthy COVID-19 trials

- COVID-19 is a symptomatic condition resulting from severe acute respiratory syndrome, SARS-CoV-2, infection. Unknown until early 2020, it caused a pandemic. Given its recency and the priority given to the accurate documentation of COVID-19 research, it offers a suitable topic for calculating the proportion of untrustworthy trials with the possibility of objective estimation.
- Numerator: Taking trial retraction as a measure of integrity flaw, the Retraction Watch database identified six COVID-19 trials in July 2022 (retractionwatch.com). Note that a retraction may be the result of honest error, not misconduct.
- Denominator: A contemporaneous PubMed search (ncbi.nlm.nih.gov/PubMed), capturing citations to COVID-19 trials showed a total of 1,557 records.
- The proportion: 6/1557 = 0.4% (95% confidence interval 0.2%–0.8%) or 4 (2–8) in 1000.
- Critics might comment that the Retraction Watch database only represents the tip of the iceberg, underestimating the numerator, and leaving the proportion too low. Other critics might argue that the PubMed search underestimates the denominator, leaving the proportion too high. PubMed only indexes around 5,200 biomedical journals. According to the Scientific, Technical and Medical (STM) publishers report, there are around 48,000 journals globally, and, of these, around a third (around 16,000) are biomedical journals. So, the PubMed denominator only captures a proportion of all biomedical journals, and so it is unlikely to contribute to a low estimation of proportion. Additionally, it is important to recognize that when the numerator is not fully a part of the denominator what we get is a ratio, not a proportion. The situation here (numerator source: Retraction Watch; denominator source: PubMed) is similar to the calculation of maternal mortality ratio (numerator: maternal death; denominator: live births).

Source: DOI: 10.1002/ijgo.14837.

Self-regulation, predatory publishing, and paper mills

According to the Scientific, Technical, and Medical (STM) publishers report, there were approximately 10,000 publishers publishing respectively about 35,000 and 13,000 English- and non-English-language scientific journals. The numbers have been steadily growing. Around a third of the total are biomedical journals. These are the ones that publish trials. Throughout this book, the term journal refers to the biomedical journals group. Journals compete with each other in rankings based on citation metrics, e.g., impact factor, *h*-index, and other variants, that weight citations against the number of articles published.

Journals tend to be a self-regulating community for the majority of the global jurisdictions. They take their code of practice typically from organizations that they have developed and funded. The International Committee of Medical Journal Editors (ICMJE), the World Association of Medical Editors (WAME), and the Committee on Publication Ethics (COPE) are some familiar names. Without a legal regulatory function, these are, for all practical purposes, toothless organizations. The recent proliferation of predatory journals, paper mills, and fake peer reviews demonstrates a gaping hole in the functionality of this self-regulation.

Publishing is a multibillion-dollar trade and within it, in the absence of much formal regulation, there are the fraudsters who want to take a pie of the cake. Traditionally the publishing business charged subscribers, individuals as well as institutions. Authors who submitted papers to journals did not have to pay, but they handed over the copyright to the publishers who charged readers. As the dissemination of scientific results, produced largely through public funding, went behind a private paywall, this was considered inherently unfair. How could it be right that first the public pays for undertaking research and then it pays again for accessing its findings? The business model changed as the open access publication agenda took hold. Funders of research became prepared to pay what is known as the article processing charges for publication so that research findings could be immediately publicly accessed. The copyright arrangements changed as various levels of open access emerged including the permissions for unrestricted reuse. It opened the possibility for anyone to access, read, download, and even distribute published results of trials without any financial or legal barrier. This all happened at the same time as the world turned digital.

Today an active trialists' daily reality includes receiving unsolicited emails that invite them to submit papers promising fast turnaround times. There may be associated invitations to take part in journals as editors. These likely originate from predatory journals that exploit the

Institution: A clinical academic organization such as a university or a hospital, where trials take place. Institutions have primary responsibility for the ethical and professional conduct of their trials.

International Committee of Medical Journal Editors (ICMJE): Provides guidance to journals on publishing policies such as uniform requirements for manuscripts (icmje.org).

World Association of Medical Editors (WAME): Aims to improve editorial standards through self-regulation (wame.org).

Committee on Publication Ethics (COPE): Issues guidance to journals on publishing policies. (publicationethics.org)

Open access publication: Open knowledge dissemination via free-of-cost availability of research outputs and journal articles online.

open access publication model to unscrupulously make money. They ask authors to pay the article processing charge, something that legitimate open access journals also do. Of course, this is the same charge that when applied in good faith makes open access publication possible for genuine research dissemination. Depending on the amount of payment at the top end, there is immediate open access to the version of the record of the article that comes with all singing, all dancing as published formally by the journal (gold open access) or there are cheaper options including self-archiving by authors of their preprints or accepted manuscripts before copy editing possibly with an embargo period introducing some delay in open access (green open access). The future may see the development of legitimate academic-led publishing initiatives that are free and immediately open access (diamond open access). Alongside the Guccis and Armanis in this market, are the bogus brands. The former are listed in the Directory of Open Access Journals (DOAJ) or the Open Access Scholarly Publishers Association (OASPA). The bogus brands take advantage of the digital platforms that look virtually identical to the listed journals, including genuine-looking impact factors, indexing, ISSNs (International Standard Serial Numbers), DOIs (Digital Object Identifiers), and more. They may even list established, known academics as members of their editorial boards without permission. Thus, the brand identity takes a form very similar to that of a genuine scientific publisher. Indeed, some have even fooled the experts and have probably even entered into the recognized listings produced by known legitimate publishers.

Predatory journals approach authors indiscriminately and offer quick publication. They can easily entice naive trialists to part with their money in return for a publication that would not be processed in the standard fashion. There will be little or no peer review. The standard peer review is not the best game in town (see below), but certainly, it is not bogus. The notification of article processing charges is usually not upfront. If on discovery of having fallen prey trialists wish to withdraw, they are usually threatened with legal notices and demands for damages. Genuine trials may thus be lost to these scams. To prevent this wastage one suggestion is that legitimate journals should offer the possibility of duplicate publication something that is facilitated if the predatory journal does not seek a copyright agreement. Box 7.2 gives an approach to distinguish between genuine and predatory publishing, pointing towards some warning signs that may or may not be sufficiently discriminatory.

A related problem is that of paper mills, paying someone to buy authorship on a pre-written paper that is likely to be plagiarized and fabricated. When predatory journals meet the paper mills, the bogus assessment process replaces that standard peer review, and the prospect grows of many more irresponsibly published trials. We are at this crossroads

Funder: Organizations such as governmental agencies, philanthropists, research charities, and industries that provide funding for a trial under contract to an institution.

Predatory publishing: Journals publishing irresponsibly, putting financial interest ahead of the trustworthiness of the scientific record.

Version of record: The final published version of the manuscript in its definitive form with copyediting and typesetting completed, metadata applied, and DOI (digital object identifier) allocated.

Preprint: A publicly posted draft version of a manuscript. usually simultaneously posted at the first submission to a journal, and is available prior to completion of its formal peer review. Preprints usually have DOIs (Digital Object Identifiers) and can be cited like other any other paper.

Box 7.2: Comparison of genuine *versus* predatory publishing

Warning signs	Subscription journals	Open access journals	Predatory journals
● Funding the research published*	No	No	No
● Article processing charge to authors or their institutions or funders	No	Yes	Yes
● Subscription fees to institutions and readers	Yes	No	Perhaps
● Charging both authors and readers	No	No	Perhaps
● Notification of charges upfront	Yes	Yes	No
● Editorial and peer review process compliant with some standard, e.g., COPE	Yes	Yes	No or unclear
● Editors few and with unknown affiliations	No	No	Yes
● Papers per issue usually few	No	No	Yes
● Journal full address unavailable	No	No	Yes
● Unknown metrics and indices	No	No	Yes

Some funders have their own journals to publish the research they fund.
Source: DOI's: 10.1186/s12916-020-01566-1; 10.24318/cope.2019.3.6.

just now. More importantly, paper mills have successfully penetrated the genuine publishing business, even organizing fake peer reviews of fake papers on an industrial scale. Preferred reviewers suggested by such authors tend to have non-attributable email addresses, turn around their assessments very quickly with positive but brief comments, and recommend acceptance. This pattern is repeated submission after submission. Traditional publishers have only recently become wise to this and have established a multistakeholder consensus over how to address this problem (united2act.org). This will require detective work, researching the paper mills industry, and developing of automated tools using Artificial Intelligence (AI), for example, to help verify author and reviewer identities. The peer reviewer databases too need to be cleared of the fabricated contact details. Sadly, as the assessment of fake peer review is itself imperfect, there is a possibility that some genuine trials may be lost as the publishers attempt to clean the pollution resulting from the inclusion of milled papers. Post-publication scientific record correction is a mandatory part of the strategy. Journals have started to retract papers thought to have been accepted for publication because of manipulation of their standard assessment process.

Paper mills:
The business of publishing fake research papers and selling authorship.

Fake peer review:
A form of publication process manipulation where fabricated contact details are supplied in the preferred peer reviewer list to journals at the time of submission, and then positive reviews are supplied from these fabricated addresses.

Publishing trials responsibly could mean many things. One aspiration, for example, could be that all stakeholders involved in trial publishing must work toward zero-carbon emissions, something that is highly relevant for global health and well-being. But empty slogans achieve nothing. Retracted papers cannot be reused, except perhaps in researching research fraud. If salvageable, they may be republished with major corrections implemented (Chapter 10). The idea is that they should never come be published in the first place. The need to retract trials following publication no doubt will impinge on the zero-carbon aspiration. Publishing science irresponsibly will have consequences for everyone!

Peer review of trial manuscripts

Journals appoint editors and other publishing staff to organize the peer review of trial manuscripts and their publication. Journals may be said to have a gatekeeper role in that completed research goes through their hands before becoming published literature. When one learns of how insufficient and unclear journals' authors' instructions, advice to peer reviewers and research misconduct investigation policies are, the seriousness required for this role is found wanting. When it comes to peer review quality, biomedical journals are regarded as the bad apples among science journals, particularly in clinical research. Peer review is not an easy task when viewed in light of the heavy responsibility placed on the shoulders of a couple of individuals to protect the trustworthiness of the scientific record. Journals' role as custodians of published clinical evidence integrity has been tarnished by the recent scandals associated with retractions. That trust in trials has taken a nosedive is thus no surprise. The role journal editors and peer reviewers have played in this debacle requires introspection. Responsible publication, not just responsible research conduct, is now a public demand.

The high pedestal on which peer review has been placed is perhaps nothing other than a marketing or branding effort for the gatekeeper role of journals. On closer examination, the gatekeeper role of journals appears to be not much other than false pretense. By the time a completed trial manuscript lands at a journal's door, the research work has already been completed. At this late stage, there is virtually no scope left for injecting any greater scientific rigor into the completed trial through anything that a journal can do. Perhaps the manuscript language can be moderated a bit to avoid spin in writing, something that is recognized as a questionable research practice (Box 10.2). Like in all interventions, there are risks involved. Peer reviews and even journals themselves, despite guidelines against citation manipulation, are known to insist that authors include references to their own publications during manuscript revisions to boost their citation metrics such as h-index and impact factor.

Artificial Intelligence (AI): Automated solutions, using methods like machine learning, natural language processing, data mining, information retrieval, and other computer science methods, to perform tasks that usually require human intelligence. Traditional AI processes data to give results, for example, plagiarism and author identity checks can be automated.

Formal peer review: Evaluation of scientific manuscripts by others working in the same field invited by journal editors prior to acceptance for publication as definitive articles representing the version of the record.

Coercive citation practices: Peer reviews and journals may coerce authors to include references to their own papers during manuscript revisions.

Peer reviewers and editors can also misdirect trialists in methodology. It is common experience that peer reviewers ask for p-values in baseline comparisons, something that is an oxymoron. In properly randomized trials, group allocation takes place using a chance procedure (a random number generator is used, unpredictability is added via variables block size, stratification is deployed for creating groups balanced for key prognostic variables, and allocation sequence is kept concealed), so whether baseline characteristics are similar or dissimilar between the group is a matter of chance. Thus, seeking a p-value for the comparison makes no sense. In addition to this, as the p-values are related to sample size, in a small trial with considerable baseline imbalance, the statistical significance test could fail (false negative) and, conversely, in a large trial without baseline imbalance, a negligible difference could show up as being statistically significant (false positive). Journal editors uncritically expect authors to follow the misguided advice given by peer reviewers on statistical testing for baseline characteristics. Given the power editors exercise over authors, they are known to concede while muttering, "I am including the p-value although it is not considered good practice in baseline data." Thus, formal peer review is a double-edged sword. It cut both ways. Unfortunately, it is blunt when it attempts to cut one way (peer reviewers lack resources and competence in offering guidance to authors) and it has negative consequences when it cuts the other way (peer reviewers may offer misguided advice that goes unchecked in the hands of the editors).

Some journals ask peer reviewers to examine "fit" for the journal, comment on plagiarism, and check the grammar. These are not really the kind of tasks in which peer review expertise should be needed for. The "fit" should be assessed by editors. The latter two issues, in the current age, are best addressed by assistive tools powered by AI. In the case of grammar checking, the native language of most peer reviewers is not English so their comments in this regard are likely to be misplaced. Apart from the above, all that is left is for editors and peer reviewers is to crosscheck that the trial took place as prospectively registered. Even this relatively simple task of comparing the publicly available registration and the manuscript submitted seems to go wrong in the hands of journals. Have a look at the case study in Box 7.3. Crosschecking what is reported against the approved protocol and the statistical analysis plan is a more effortful task (see case study in Box 2.6). The part played by the failure of the editorial and peer review oversight system in misreported trials is recognized in the corrective efforts required via campaigns such as AllTrials and RIAT as well as the post-publication voluntary reviews undertaken by sleuths. The editorial and peer review assignments concerning crosschecks against publicly available trial records might be done better via

Power: The ability to influence others. The role asymmetry in a relationship permits the powerful to influence the vulnerable. The responsibility to prevent influence from turning into abuse lies with the powerful party.

AllTrials: A campaign for all past and present clinical trials to be registered and their methods and summary results reported (alltrials.net).

RIAT: An international effort to Restoring Invisible and Abandoned (unpublished and misreported) trials (restoringtrials.org).

Data sleuthing: Post-publication investigation of possible research misconduct and questionable research practices by volunteer researchers.

Box 7.3: Case study–A 2023 retraction of a 2022 trial

- The ICMJE made prospective registration a requirement for publication in mid-2005. An evaluation over a decade after this directive found that only around four of every 10 trials published in PubMed journals in 2018 were prospectively publicly registered.
- A 2022 publication of a trial reported that it obtained human research ethics committee approval, which was publicly registered.
- The trial registration document has been publicly available since mid-2020.
- The trial manuscript was with the journal in its assessment system for around 10 weeks from submission to acceptance according to the publication history reported.
- Within a few months of the trial publication, it was retracted at the request of the editor-in-chief and the executive editor.
- The 2023 retraction notice stated the reason for retraction as follows: "After publication, we were made aware of discrepancies between the trial registration and the published paper. No relevant changes to the protocol/registration were noted and deviations from the protocol were not described within the paper. What was published is, in effect, a different trial to that described in the trial registration...."
- The retraction notice ended as follows: "Apologies are offered to the readers of the journal that discrepancies between the trial registration and the published paper were not detected during the peer review process."
- The reason for the failure to detect the discrepancies between the registration and the submitted manuscript during the journal's assessment, and the fate of the trial following its retraction remain unknown at the time of drafting this book.

Sources: DOI's: 10.1016/j.ijnurstu.2022.104387; 10.1016/j.ijnurstu.2023.104558; 10.1136bmj.m982.

automated tools developed using traditional AI and, in the near future, these checks may become so proficient that they may even replace human input.

The use of generative AI for peer review is a different matter as it puts confidentiality at risk and, at present, it is error-prone. For now, ICMJE recommends that peer reviewers should seek permission from journals if they wish to use AI in the review of manuscripts. As the majority of peer reviewers work for nothing under heavy time pressures and the task of evaluating research integrity is effortful, the chance of obtaining a competent assessment even from well-intentioned souls is quite low. The reality is that the expertise required for performing an in-depth assessment is not widely or readily available. Plagiarism in peer review reports is another recently recognized problem. As journals tend to keep peer-reviewers' identities and their reports secret, this may serve as a hidden incentive for them to plagiarise text. Sources similar to the manuscript being evaluated can be readily picked up by searching the literature and then the text can be copied and pasted into the peer review report.

Research integrity: Undertaking trials in accordance with ethical and professional principles and standards. Integrity failures may result from honest errors or deliberate misconduct. Responsible research conduct paves the way for trial methods and findings to be regarded as trustworthy.

Integrity appraisal of trial manuscripts

The typical questions asked of manuscripts received by editors and peer reviewers are: Is it new? Is it true? Is it noteworthy? These questions are asked sequentially.

Journals' obsession with novelty is quite strange as replication, a recognized scientific virtue, should not be forgotten. Trials may justifiably be replicated whenever previously evaluated effects of interventions need reassessment in a different setting or in a different participant group or with some modification to the intervention, etc. Moreover, whether something is novel cannot really be considered until one can be sure that the findings are likely to be true. Why put the cart before the horse? The cart that carries the message from the trial will be pulled by the strength of the horse based on the trial's integrity and quality. So, the analogy of putting the cart before the horse captures the problem arising from doing things in the wrong order well. Chapter 2 proposed a new critical appraisal where it is recommended that the starting point in a trial's assessment should be the examination of research integrity. This would be a suitable approach for editors and peer reviewers to follow too. Once integrity screening has taken place (Box 7.4), it is possible to move to whether the findings address a priority problem and whether they are valid (unbiased) and precise. In addition, the incorporation of pragmatism features in the trial design and analysis will maximize trial usefulness for application in the healthcare setting (Box 2.5).

How confident can we be in assessing trial integrity? This is another challenging question that needs research investment. The integrity tests proposed in Box 7.4 have not so far been scientifically assessed for their

Usefulness of trials: A multidimensional concept, evaluating integrity, research priority, pragmatism, validity, and precision.

Research priority: The ranking or selection of a few among the many established research gaps and needs.

Research gap: A gap in knowledge.

Research need: A research gap resulting in an inability to make healthcare decisions.

Pragmatism: The extent to which trials can be anticipated to produce useful results to directly inform healthcare practice and policy.

Box 7.4: Proposed screening for randomized clinical trial integrity

Domains	Proposed integrity tests	Features of concern
Submission	• Cover letter • Preferred reviewers • Request for information or data	• Cover letter missing, paper title mismatch, or text similar to other submissions received. • Author's email address similar to preferred reviewers' address. • Author and reviewer internet protocol or IP address same. • Absence of response or unusual responses to requests for details by journal.

Title page	● Author details	● Name and email address mismatch. ● Changes requested without justification. ● Author numbers are not congruent with trial size or effort.
Methods and results	● Ethics committee approval ● Registration ● Statistical methods ● Recruitment ● Losses to follow-up ● Participant characteristics ● Effects reported	● Approval missing ● Registration missing, not prospective, or not in a recognized platform. ● Missing hospital city and region details. ● Methods text generic or not matching trial objective. ● Missing protocol and statistical analysis plan or with parts redacted without explanation or justification. ● Missing reporting checklist. ● Issues with numbers in the trial participant flow diagram. ● Mismatch in reported statistics and independent calculations. ● Implausible results not explained by the play of chance.
Statements	● Acknowledgment ● Conflicts of interest declaration (financial and personal) ● Funding disclosure (direct support given for undertaking the trial)	● Wording unusual, awkward, or in a style different from the manuscript text. ● Undeclared conflicts of interest.

The above is not a complete list.
Source: DOI's: 10.1016/j.jclinepi.2022.07.006; 10.1016/j.jclinepi.2024.111365.

performance through a systematic approach to measurement for accurately categorizing the observations made when raising integrity concerns. The need to distinguish between a trial feature that may point toward bias or toward an integrity flaw is all too important. For example, in relation to attrition bias, a reduction in missing outcome data is desired (Box 2.2). However, could the complete absence of missing data be a marker of an integrity flaw? Similarly, the financial ties of authors with manufacturers are associated with positive findings in trials, but is this a marker of bias or that of an integrity flaw? These questions have not so far been addressed scientifically. For undeclared conflicts of financial interests, have a look at a relevant case study in Box 7.5.

Box 7.5: Case study–Failure to declare financial conflicts of interest

- Surgical mesh to treat uterine prolapse or stress urinary incontinence has been a controversial topic.
- When trialists receive industry funding there is a higher likelihood of positive findings being reported in trials, suggesting the possibility of bias arising due to financial ties (DOI: 10.1136/bmj.i6770).
- A 2024 evidence synthesis examined if clinical investigators in the USA contributing as authors to articles published on surgical mesh in peer-reviewed journals declared industry funding.
- Relevant articles were identified through a PubMed search (2014–2021) and data were extracted from them regarding authors' declarations of conflicts of interests.
- Industry funding given to the physician authors within one year of their paper's publication was identified through the publicly available CMS Open Payments database (openpaymentsdata.cms.gov).
- There were 247 clinical investigators in the USA contributing as authors in the relevant articles. Of these 149 authors had received payments (> $100) while 98 authors had not.
- Of those who did not receive payments, 81 authors (83%) correctly declared a lack of conflict.
- Of the authors who had received payments, 20 (13%) did not make a declaration. Surprisingly, 101 authors (68%) explicitly declared no financial conflict of interest but had received payments. The undeclared amounts were $100–1,000 (54, 36%), $1,000–10,000 (36, 24%), $10,000–100,000 (20, 13%), and >$100,000 (11, 7%).
- The review concluded that journals' guidelines regarding the declaration of the author's financial conflicts of interest were not being followed.

Declarations of financial conflicts of interest are distinct from funding disclosures as the latter pertains to transparently stating the direct support given for undertaking research.
Source: DOI: 10.1186/s41073-024-00145-9.

The judicious application of integrity tests to trial manuscripts is hampered not just by the scarcity of integrity test performance studies, but also by an absence of objective data concerning the prevalence of flawed trials (Box 7.1) and a lack of consensus over a gold standard for verifying the presence or absence of integrity concerns. The latter is required for establishing criterion validity, i.e., for integrity test accuracy studies which will establish the level of true and false positive and negative results. False allegations are serious both for false-positives (allegations of misconduct when the trial is genuine) and false-negatives (a trial with integrity flaw passed as genuine). For trialists, false findings will affect careers and reputations. For healthcare, both false-positive and false-negative integrity test results are potentially harmful in two ways: Patients may be deprived of the benefits of useful interventions as false positive test results risk removing genuine evidence that could inform practice, or they may be exposed to risky or ineffective interventions as false negative test results permit the continued use of flawed evidence. The purpose of pointing this out is to highlight the current limitations in dealing objectively with concerns about trial integrity and to point the way towards the research-based solutions required to address this issue. The trial integrity appraisals once scientifically evaluated for their level of performance will serve journals in screening trials ahead of publication and will also help reviewers in filtering trials being considered for inclusion in evidence syntheses (Chapter 9). Automation will no doubt develop alongside to help undertake trial manuscript screening.

Journals' instructions to authors

Trialists announce what they are going to do, tell publicly how it is going as they do it, and finally say what they have found according to what they said they were going to do and what they did. Journals tell this story.

Authors' instructions is where trialists begin their interaction with journals. Here the trialist would be expected to find what ought to be reported. Indeed, some may even design and conduct trials in a way so as to meet these reporting requirements. Systematic evaluations of authors' instructions in journals have found deficiencies in important areas such as ethics committee approval, funding disclosure, declaration of conflicts of interests, data sharing, authorship, etc. Specification of the requirements for trials by journals is fundamental to publishing trials responsibly.

A reporting checklist, i.e., a minimum list of information required for writing manuscripts, is frequently used by authors and deployed by journals. For trials, CONSORT is there as a prominent checklist among the authors' instructions issued by many journals. There are also the SPIRIT, GRIPP, SAGER, DELTA and TIDieR reporting checklists relevant to trials. It is important to recognize that reporting checklists are not synonymous with methodological guidance. Poorly designed and conducted trials may meet all the reporting checklist items. The reporting checklists are also not a replacement for authors' instructions which should be crafted by journals specifying their requirements for trials.

The Transparency and Openness Promotion (TOP) guidelines are a step in the right direction for journals. TOP offers an outline of generic standards for reporting based on open science principles. The standards need specification for application in trial publication practice, focusing on prospective registration, protocol publication, complete reporting with respect to trial conduct, statistical analysis plan preregistration, data and

EQUATOR: A network for improving health research reporting (equator-network. org). Trials benefit from:

SPIRIT: Standard Protocol Items: Recommendations for Interventional Trials.

CONSORT: Consolidated Standards of Reporting Trials.

GRIPP: Guidance for Reporting Involvement of Patients and the Public.

SAGER: A checklist for gender-sensitive reporting.

DELTA: A checklist for reporting the sample size calculation in trials

TIDieR: Template for Intervention Description and Replication.

analytic code sharing, as well as promotion of replication trials. A proposal is sketched out in Box 7.6. Using these standards, journals can enforce and encourage trialists to comply with open science practices to varying degrees. For example, ICMJE mandates prospective registration (Chapter 5) and data sharing plans for trials. The former is enforced but the latter is an encouragement. ICMJE currently only requires trial registration to include data sharing plans and the published article to include a statement about it. However, it does not go as far as the ideal, which is to share the analyzable dataset (derived from the raw data) properly deidentified in accordance with privacy laws. This limits the opportunity to undertake independent data integrity checks and replication of reported results. Trialists and journals don't have to wait for ICMJE to issue a further directive on data sharing. They can just leap forward now to actual data sharing (see below). Instead of restricting themselves to making the data available on request, authors should provide it on manuscript submission. Journals can reward compliance with open science practices, e.g., by publishing trial papers with badges to signal whenever there is data sharing (Box 7.6).

TOP: Guidelines for Transparency and Openness Promotion (TOP) in journal policies and practices (osf.io/ud578).

Box 7.6: Proposals for the specification of instructions to authors for journals to publish trials responsibly

Open science standard	Lip service	Full compliance in trial publication
Trial preregistration	Journal merely requires article to state that there has been registration	Prospective registration date and link plus ethics committee approval are verified by the journal and provided in the article
Design and analysis reporting	Journal encourages design and analysis transparency in its authors' instructions	Journal enforces adherence to design transparency standards via its review and the article appends the approved dated protocol unredacted with trial oversight documentation as well as any modifications to protocol reported in methods
Analysis plan preregistration	Journal merely seeks a statement on whether or not an *a priori* statistical analysis plan exists	The *a priori* statistical analysis plan registration date and link are verified by the journal and the article appends it in unredacted form with any modifications reported in methods
Analysis code transparency	Journal merely seeks a statement on whether or not the analysis code is available	Journal reproduces the analysis using the code provided during its review and the article appends the code or provides a link to a trusted repository verified before publication
Data transparency	Journal merely seeks a statement on whether or not the dataset of the reported analysis is available	Data posted to a trusted repository, journal seeks a certificate of verification of data integrity and reproduces independently the reported analyses using the shared dataset before publication
Data citation	Journal merely seeks a statement on whether or not the analysis dataset of the reported is available	Article is not published without appropriate citation for the shared dataset posted to a trusted repository and the publication is badged
Replication	Journal says nothing or does not actively discourage submission of replication trials by explicitly demanding novelty	Journal invites trial protocols as a submission option for replication trials with peer review prior to trial completion or without knowledge of the repeat trial results
Contributorship	Journal merely seeks that authorship criteria are met and those with conflicts of interests make declarations	Journal enforces that all authors and those acknowledged provide contributor roles and make declarations about both financial and personal conflicts of interests

Proposals and open data badge from Transparency and Openness Promotion (TOP) guidelines (osf.io/ud578).
See Box 3.3 for an open science vision for randomized clinical trials.
See Box 5.1 for an outline of a trial protocol recommending design-specific reporting checklists.
See Box 5.3 for an outline of a statistical analysis plan for a trial.
See Box 6.2 for a proposal for a trial's complete and contemporaneous public documentation.
See Box 8.2 for Contributor Roles Taxonomy (CRediT) system classifying the roles played by individual authors and those acknowledged in a trial publication (DOI:10.1087/20150211).

Data sharing

Healthcare research is undertaken for societal benefit. Going beyond the published trial results, data sharing maximizes the trial benefits for the public good, something that is a feature of the risk-benefit assessment in the ethics committee approval (Chapter 4). Since 2018–19, the ICMJE requirements pertaining to data are restricted to making a data sharing plan public at the time of prospective registration and then making a data sharing statement in the publication of the trial results without any formal requirement to publicly share the data. This is partly because secrecy, not transparency, has been the norm in the healthcare research culture. This leaves it open for trialists to specify data access criteria defeating the real purpose of data sharing. Hopefully, this is going to change soon for trials.

Let's take the example of space science, a discipline comprising astronomy and astrophysics as well as solar, planetary and lunar sciences. Active data archives provide live access to researchers, and in specific cases to the general public too. This means that all space science data gathered are accessible without secrecy. There may be some reasonable restrictions applied but open data is the norm, as is open access publication. Okay, space science is not healthcare research; perhaps healthcare research has not been so technologically advanced. However, today there is no technical barrier as to why trials cannot be open just as space science is. The TOP guidelines are pushing for this to happen (Box 7.6).

Recommendations for responsible data sharing in trials are being put forward for stakeholder organizations to implement, maximizing the benefits while minimizing the risks. Perhaps data privacy issues are the key risk that ethics committees and consenting participants would want to be reassured about. Participants give informed consent to share their data with the proviso that their confidentiality and privacy will be protected. The patient information prepared to accompany the informed consent should give details of how this will be ensured (Box 4.4). Data deindentification or anonymization is now a well-developed technique. The greatest resistance to data sharing probably comes from trialists themselves as they want to protect the data for secondary analyses to be undertaken by themselves or with their input. If they made all that effort to properly collect data, why should they just give it away to others? For addressing this concern, there is a need to think beyond the trial in terms of data stewardship, i.e., reaping the fruits of the trial effort through the continuing use of the accompanying digital asset created.

Trials undertaken for regulatory approval are not covered in this book. Still, beyond an initial embargo period placed for safeguarding intellectual property and commercially sensitive information, data sharing remains a feasible option. Even if the commercial trials don't publicly share

Regulator A formal body set up: for official approvals of medicines and devices, e.g., Food and Drug Administration (FDA), European Medicines Agency (EMA), etc.

data, it is possible to seek this information from regulators to whom the data have been submitted for approval (Box 2.6). This is possible as openness in governmental policies, activities and decisions is enshrined in law. The regulatory responsibility includes the obligation to provide public access to the official documents produced or received on written request. When making decisions about disclosure regulators take into account any binding confidentiality agreements, privacy protection requirements, etc. Whenever an overriding societal interest can be established, regulators could engage in disclosure of the trial data they have in their possession. Thus, in the foreseeable future, data sharing could become a part and parcel of the official regulatory approval process.

For trials outside the regulatory framework, all stakeholder organizations must commit. This is necessary because the long-term aspect of data sharing requires that institutions establish a sustainable infrastructure for data custodianship, ensuring that data are findable, accessible, interoperable and reusable. Funders should work with institutions to make this a reality. For data sharing to work, its technical aspects would need to be attended to in detail, e.g., analyzable datasets are derived from raw data and upon sharing are analyzable only when accompanied by metadata describing the dataset. Journals should ensure that the data sharing statement at the time of publication of findings should come with the citation of the dataset posted on a trusted repository.

Data sharing will allow reanalysis to independently examine if the reported results can be replicated, something that journals should implement even if initially the data are not publicly shared. This should help reduce the risk of misconduct allegations. Moreover, in case of such allegations, data access will permit proper investigations. For example, anomalies such as duplicated data in multiple rows or columns, copy-pasted data, non-sequential randomization dates, etc. can all be picked up and concerns of this nature can be readily eliminated. It is possible the data access option will convert potential complaints into scientific enquiries. This is important because whenever an integrity concern is raised about a trial, such investigations are stressful and time-consuming for innocent trialists and costly for all parties involved without data access. Data sharing will help in evidence synthesis, particularly in meta-analysis where it will become feasible to perform more sophisticated, more statistically powerful re-analyses combining many trial datasets (Chapter 9). Other secondary analyses of the data shared will help advance new scientific hypotheses not originally framed as part of the trial and perhaps there will be studies undertaken within several trials addressing questions not addressable within a single trial alone. For example, subgroups effects not evaluable within individual trials could be explored in evidence syntheses through individual participant data (IPD) meta-

FAIR: Data sharing acronym describing the notion that data should be Findable, Accessible, Interoperable and Reusable.

Statistical power: The ability to statistically reject the null hypothesis when it is indeed false. Power is related to sample size and the number of outcomes in the comparison groups. The larger the sample size, the more the power, the narrower the confidence interval around the effect of the intervention, and the lower is the risk that a possible effect could be missed due to the play of chance.

Individual participant data (IPD) meta-analysis: A statistical synthesis that uses participant-level data collected in the trials included in a systematic review to produce a powerful summary result.

analysis using the datasets combined (Box 9.2). The manuscripts using these existing trial datasets would need to cite them correctly giving credit to the original trialists.

The now well-recognized greater public good that emerges from data sharing ought to catapult the trialist community into taking action, converting their plans and statements into actual sharing within a reasonable timeframe after trial completion. This can happen through voluntary action without the need to wait for the formal requirements mandated by journals. More importantly, data sharing should be seen as part of the timely and complete public documentation of the trial outlined in Chapters 5 and 6.

Openness in the publication process

Journals have the responsibility to ensure that manipulation of the publication process in any form does not take place. Fake peer review is an example of journals becoming victims of deception due to external intervention. However, in peer review, there are also many internal difficulties, e.g., unauthorized use of information gained through reviewing activities, confidentiality violation through disclosure of reviewed information to others, etc. This is in part the result of the single-blind nature of traditional peer review where the identities of the reviewers are deliberately kept hidden from authors and readers by journals. Only the editors see their reports. Double-blinding peer review, proposed in some research fields, is illogical for trials; it makes no sense to blind peer reviewers from trial prospective registration details. So how can one counter the power imbalance created by single-blind peer review? In this regard, open peer review including naming peer reviewers (open identities) with the publishing of peer review reports and authors' responses alongside articles (open reports) is preferable over the traditional blind peer review system. Peer reviewers too should be asked to make public their declarations of conflicts of interests in the same way as authors are required to do for transparency. The open peer review reports should be assigned a DOI, making them fully citable.

Going forward, with prospective registration, protocol publication and availability of *a priori* statistical analysis plan, the transparency achieved in the course of the trial should continue in the publication process. Alongside trial manuscript submission to a journal, it is feasible to make the trial findings public through the publication of preprints, which are available for peer review by anyone (open pre-review). The publicly provided comments on preprints can be put together with those received via the formal peer review organized by the journal. If the formal peer review using the open identities and open reports formats is live

Publication process manipulation: Misconduct in the publication process, e.g., organization of or taking part in fake peer review, unauthorized use of information gained through peer reviewing activities, and confidentiality violation through disclosure of peer reviewed information to others.

Open peer review: Evaluation of scientific manuscripts by journals in keeping with open science principles whereby peer review reports and authors' responses are published alongside accepted articles. By contrast, in traditional peer review reviewer identity and their reports are kept blind.

or contemporaneous, this has various advantages. In case the manuscript is accepted, the revision can incorporate all the changes required in one go. On the other hand, if the manuscript is rejected or if it is withdrawn, the comments given will remain publicly available. This is especially relevant if the comments raise integrity concerns; authors will not be able to keep these concerns hidden from the journal to whom they make the resubmission. Making manuscripts publicly available from day one of submission and also making peer review reports and editors' comments available open in the publication process has advantages over the traditional confidential and secretive process. Journals, e.g., F1000Research and eLife, have started to move towards this level of openness.

Chapter 7: Publishing trials responsibly – Key points

Execution of trials (advice to trialists)

- Conduct and report the trial so as to meet responsible publication requirements based on Transparency and Openness Promotion (TOP) guidelines.
- Provide publicly date-time-stamped prospective registration before the first participant is enrolled and *a priori* statistical analysis plan before the follow up of the last participant is completed. Data sharing plan should be included in the prospective registration.
- Go beyond the current data sharing requirement for a statement in the trial manuscript. Share the deidentified analyzable dataset derived from the raw data prepared in compliance with privacy laws. It should be accompanied by metadata and sited in a secure repository.
- Seek badges for compliance with TOP standards such as prospective registration and data sharing according to the policy of the journal.
- Engage actively in communications about the manuscript and its review whether officially organized by your chosen journal or provided via unsolicited comments, e.g., comments on the preprint and published conference abstract or poster.
- Take care to avoid a predatory publisher. Never use a paper mill.
- Never engage in manipulation of peer review. If you must provide a preferred reviewers list ensure that they are not your past

Transparency in research: Open research practices including prospective registration, adherence to trial design, *a priori* statistical analysis plan, data sharing, and timely and complete public reporting.

co-authors, nor geographically based anywhere near you, your trial collaborators or your institutions.

- After trial completion, i.e., after primary outcome data collection from the last randomized participant, post the main results on the registry within 12 months. Submit the manuscript to a journal within this timeframe in the hope of getting the trial results formally published in a definitive article (version of record created with its own DOI) within 24 months of trial completion.
- Publish a preprint at the same time when first submitting the trial manuscript to a journal. Most journals provide this option at the time of submission of the manuscript. Preprints are not considered prior publication, so they are not disqualifiers for submission to a journal. Preprints usually have DOI's and can be cited like any other paper. The preprint version is updated with a link to the final published version.

Conflicts of interest: Potential or perceived compromise in the objectivity or judgement of anyone involved in research and publication due to financial or personal (non-financial) interests. Failure of declaration is considered research misconduct.

Writing tips for trial authors

- See related key points in Chapters 5 and 6.
- **Title:** Provide the correct details according to the journal's instructions. Follow the authorship integrity principles (Chapter 8).
- **Abstract:** Write according to reporting checklists. Give prospective registration details.
- **Introduction:** The trial justification, both ethical and scientific, should be provided as essential background (Chapter 4).
- **Methods and results:** Write according to the reporting checklist. Give prospective registration details and a link to the *a priori* statistical analysis plan. Give data sharing details.
- **Tables and figures:** Provide flow charts giving participant flow as observed in the trial including a complete description of losses. Write titles for tables and figures in sufficient detail to permit them to stand alone without the need to refer to the main text. Give detailed footnotes.
- **Discussion:** Place the trial findings in the context of existing literature providing a detailed explanation for any outlying observations. Provide an updated evidence synthesis (Chapter 9).
- **Data sharing statement:** Ensure this is as open as possible, respecting the privacy laws. Prepare the deidentified or anonymized data analysis file on which the shared statistical analytic codes can be applied. There should be a citation to the trusted repository where the dataset has been posted.
- **Funding disclosures:** Given full account of direct funding to the trial.

- **Conflicts of interest:** Declare conflicts of (both financial and personal) interests of trialists, citizens involved in trial co-production, and independent members of trial steering and data monitoring committees.
- **References:** Take care not to cite retracted papers or those with expressions of concerns. Do not cite papers published in predatory journals. If such citations are necessary, give the citation status (e.g., retracted) in the text as well as in the bibliography and justify the use of the citation.
- **Supplementary material:** Share statistical analysis code and output. Provide an integrity checklist in addition to any reporting checklists.

Roles of institutions, funders, and journals

- Institutions, funders and journals should implement TOP guidelines (see Box 7.6), specifying what is required for trials.
- Institutions, funders and journals should harmonize policies and procedures for research misconduct related to unethical publication practices, e.g., buying authorship through a paper mill, predatory publishing, etc., and publication process manipulation, e.g., organizing fake peer reviews, sharing peer-reviewed information with others, coercive citation practices, etc.
- Institutions, funders, journals and other stakeholders in trial conduct and publishing must work toward zero carbon emissions. Avoiding research waste is a key priority in this regard.
- Institutions and funders should implement an academic assessment system that values research integrity underpinned by transparency and data sharing, instead of putting staff under pressure to publish or perish.
- Funders should develop contracts with institutions making prospective registration and data sharing a condition of funding trials. They should prioritize research into the validation of trial integrity assessment instruments and automation of their use. The establishment of an integrity 'gold' standard for verification of trial integrity flaws and estimation of the prevalence of these flaws is required.
- Journals should have updated trial-specific authors' instructions. Prevention is better than cure: Journals should publish trials responsibly, investing in proper prepublication assessment so as to minimize subsequent complaints, investigation and retraction risk (Chapter 10). They should implement research integrity training programmes for their staff and should routinely

Inadequate citation practices: Erroneous citations in published articles. These may include unnecessary self-citation as well as citations of works of others that are inappropriate, misleading,missing, inaccurate, etc.

Societies are non-profit organizations that seek to further a particular healthcare profession and the interests of their patients.

Publish or perish: An academic culture in which institutions value the numbers of papers rather than their quality or their impact.

use integrity checklists in their trial manuscript assessments in addition to screening manuscripts for plagiarism and image manipulation, using automated checks if feasible. They should offer badges for compliance with TOP standards in publications of trials.

- Journals should ensure that manipulation of peer review in any form does not take place. They should retain peer-review records and editorial comments for a period of time (a 5 or 10-year period is often advised) after their assessments in case of misconduct or manipulation allegations in the future. In this regard, open peer review including naming peer reviewers (open identities) with publishing of peer review reports and authors' responses alongside articles (open reports, preferably with DOI's assigned) is preferable over the traditional blind peer review system.
- Data sharing ought to become the norm unless exceptional circumstances apply. To ensure data sharing in all trials, there is a need to provide training in data science and establish a secure infrastructure. Stakeholders organizing congresses, including professional societies, should seek data sharing details as part of conference abstracts, posters and presentations.

8 *Authorship of trials*

Authorship gives credit to those who make a substantial contribution in the design, conduct, analysis, reporting, and other critical aspects of a clinical trial. Authors are accountable for the trial in its published form. Authorship carries with it an element of prestige, and has both social and financial implications, as it plays a role in intuitional appointments and promotion systems. Collaboration is key in randomized clinical trials. Large multicenter clinical trials, with thousands of participants recruited across many countries and continents may involve hundreds of contributors. Trialists alone cannot deliver trials; site investigators, patient representatives among others help in the successful execution of trials. The International Committee of Medical Journal Editors (ICMJE) criteria are far too rigid and are unfit for clinical trials. Descriptions of contributions in the Contributor Roles Taxonomy (CRediT) are also insufficient for clinical trials. With strict adherence to rules, only a proportion of the contributors may be named in the authorship of trial publications. Pressure to publish leads to authorship abuse and disputes. Therefore, forward planning is required with a transparent, flexible, and imaginative approach to honestly attribute credit to those who make the successful completion of trials possible.

Authorship: Gives credit to those who make a substantial contribution in the design, conduct, analysis, reporting, and other critical aspects of a clinical trial. Authors are accountable for the trial in its published form.

What is there in authorship?

Journal: An establishment composed of editors and other publishing staff who organize peer reviews of trial manuscripts and their publication.

The key features of trial collaborations are: There are many contributors; each contributor brings particular knowledge, skills, or expertise to the trial's design, conduct and analysis; each contributor is an individual who holds personal views and ideas about how credit should be given for their contribution in the reporting of the trial; each individual operates within a particular setting, such as a clinic, a university, or industry; and, given that workplace cultures vary between settings, individuals experience the pressure to publish as authors not only because of their own beliefs but also because of what their institutions want from them in appointments, and in their annual appraisals for career progression and promotion. Thus, authorship is not just an academic matter, it also carries with it an element of prestige and has both social and financial implications. Authorship has the potential to become a controversial issue, a "hot potato", and it must be handled with care and attention to detail from the start.

Authorship gives credit to those who design, conduct, analyze, and report a piece of research. Authors appear on the title page of the trial manuscript and at the top of the published paper, above the trial's abstract. Importantly, authorship gives responsibility for the integrity of the

DOI: 10.1201/9781003461401-8

research published on those named as authors. Other contributors to the research are named in the acknowledgments section, usually placed at the end of the discussion section, just before the references in the published paper. In cases of queries pertaining to research integrity, accountability rests with the authors. There are set criteria for authorship (see below). Depending on the academic discipline, its culture, and traditions, adherence to the criteria fluctuates as one size cannot fit all. Therefore, variations in interpretations of authorship criteria are inevitable.

On the one hand, there are researchers who undertake the research work within the rules of their institutions; on the other, there are journals that communicate the research findings. Both institutions and journals must address the issue of authorship, though journals tend to stay at arm's length from the process leading to its determination. The journal directs queries to the named corresponding author, who should then consult other co-authors when responding. The order of authorship carries particular significance. The first author is typically the individual who has contributed most of the work, such as in designing the trial and writing the manuscript. The last author is usually someone who claims credit for supervision and tends to be the most senior or influential among the named authors. Academic cultures vary, but in general, the first and last positions, and the assignment of the corresponding author (regardless of the order in authorship), are considered the key spots in authorship. Many of the authorship disputes originate from disagreements about the order of authorship, as researchers tend to overvalue their contribution over that of other co-authors (surprisingly, the attitude tends to take the reverse form regarding accountability!). The battle for entry onto the authorship list and for the key spots within it, has the potential to "spoil the broth". Authorship order has important academic implications, as it is used as a criterion in institutional incentives systems for research staff.

The above outlines the healthcare research landscape with respect to authorship. Human randomized clinical trials, however, are different. It is important to recognize that evidence from robust trials forms the basis of effective healthcare. Multicentre trials offer the best possible avenue for achieving this. This means that varied contributions are required from many individuals. Large multi-author groups are naturally associated with multicentre trials. Some may intellectually contribute to the design, statistical analysis plan, and other methodological aspects of a trial. To realize the planned trial, the key contribution comes from clinicians who recruit and follow-up randomized participants, as without participants and outcome data, there can be no trial. Variations in the type and intensity of contributions can lead to difficulties in the assignment of authorship, especially when there are personal expectations of those who contributed, and there is pressure to publish as an author within

Institution: An academic organization that employs trialists. It focuses on research ethics and governance. Institutions tend to have their own research integrity guidelines and misconduct investigation policies, which may be deployed to address authorship disputes.

Corresponding author: The individual who is responsible for communication with the journal during the trial manuscript submission, peer review, revisions, publication, and subsequently in any post-publication correspondence.

Last author: The individual who tends to claim credit for supervision and is usually the most senior or influential amongst the authors. Note that supervision alone is not a sufficient condition for authorship.

Publish or perish: An academic culture in which institutions value the number of papers rather than their quality or their impact.

the clinical academic culture. How should trialists address this problem? There is not a ready, off-the-shelf solution.

Authorship criteria

The starting point for understanding authorship is the criteria set by the ICMJE (Box 8.1). The criteria are explicit, all must be met, and in the context of a trial, they are tough to fulfill. These criteria come with the responsibility for the integrity of the work and accountability for what is published. Unfortunately, experience shows that authorship attribution is not always strictly based on contribution. Manipulation of authorship order is also a known issue. Journals do not usually engage in detailed scrutiny with authors over how the ICMJE criteria have been met by each of the various named authors, other than seeking general assurances. If disputes arise, they tend to pass them back to the authors' employers. In some case, the disputing authors are even known to have sought the input of the courts for settling disputes through legal means.

International Committee of Medical Journal Editors (ICMJE): Has defined the criteria for authorship (icmje.org).

Generative Artificial Intelligence (AI): Can be deployed by trialists to draft and revise manuscripts, amongst other possibilities. Its use should be transparently reported without being credited in authorship.

Authorship criteria prescribed by ICMJE are difficult to fully comply with for the many who contribute to trials. The criteria are routinely flouted, and it has even been said that they are illogical and unethical. For example, highly prolific authors often appear to be guest authors, in breach of ICMJE criteria. Above all, authorship alone fails to demonstrate the contributions made by an author.

Box 8.1: Authorship criteria of the ICMJE or International Committee of Medical Journal Editors

Four recommended criteria must all be met to qualify as an author:
a. Substantial contributions to the conception or design of the work, or the acquisition, analysis, or interpretation of data for the work; and
b. Drafting the work or critically reviewing it for important intellectual content; and
c. Final approval of the version to be published; and
d. Agreement to be accountable for all aspects of the work, ensuring that questions related to the accuracy or integrity of any part of the work are appropriately investigated and resolved.

Acknowledgment
Those who do not meet all four criteria should have their contribution acknowledged. Examples of activities that alone do not qualify for authorship: Acquisition of funding, data gathering, general supervision, general administrative support, writing assistance, technical editing, language editing, and proofreading, amongst others. Use of generative Artificial Intelligence (AI) should be disclosed in acknowledgments, not included in authorship.

Source: icmje.org.

Contributorship

Contributorship, i.e., the description of contributions made by individuals in publications, has been put forward as a complementary approach to authorship. The CRediT or Contributor Roles Taxonomy system has been promoted to enable authors to provide information about individual contributions, whether the individuals are named as authors or merely acknowledged (Box 8.2). An individual contributor may have played multiple roles, and a single role may have the input from many individuals, each contributing to varying degrees. Responsibility for the accuracy of the contributions described is left to the authors. The authors' contribution statement, detailing the above, is published in the paper, usually at the end of the main text or tabulated along with the authors' names, depending on the journal's format.

> **Contributor Roles Taxonomy (CRediT):** A system for classifying the roles played by individual authors and those acknowledged in a trial publication.

An example of the authors' contribution using CRediT taken from a published trial is as follows (source: DOI: 10.1371/journal.pmed.1004 249): Contributed equally to this work: XM, FY, JW. Roles: XM (data curation, investigation, methodology), FY (data curation, investigation, methodology, writing – review and editing), JW (data curation, investigation), BX (data curation), MJ (data curation), YS (data curation), CS (data curation), YY (data curation), DX (data curation), LX (data curation), CR (data curation), CC (data curation), ZY (data curation), JL (data curation), JiL (funding acquisition, supervision, writing – review and editing, WC (data curation, funding acquisition, investigation, methodology, project administration, resources, validation, writing – original draft, writing – review and editing).

The role descriptions may also give the degree of contribution; for example, it may declare if the data curation role was equal between those named or if some took the lead. Such explicit role descriptions are on the rise. By combining the articles' Digital Object Identifier (DOI) and the unique author identifier (ORCID) with a standardized description of contributions, that is weighted, it would become possible to know exactly who contributed what and how much to each paper. This approach could pave the way for a fairer and more transparent academic assessment system, reducing the incentive for authorship abuse. Sadly, leaving the roles and contributions unclear has been far more common, or even the norm in the past.

> **ORCID:** A unique digital author identifier (orcid.org).

Box 8.2: Classification of trial roles using Contributor Roles Taxonomy (CRediT)

Roles that potentially map to ICMJE authorship criteria:
- **Conceptualization:** Formulation of ideas, research goals, aims, objectives, etc.
- **Formal analysis:** Application of statistical, mathematical, computational, or other formal techniques to analyze or synthesize data.
- **Investigation:** Conducting the trial and collecting data.
- **Methodology:** Design of the trial.
- **Review and editing of draft:** Critical review, commentary, or revision of the initial draft.
- **Writing original draft:** Preparation of the initial draft of the manuscript to be submitted for publication.

CRediT roles applicable to trials:
- **Data curation:** Management activities to annotate (producing metadata), scrub data, and maintain research data (including software code where it is necessary for interpreting the data itself) for initial use and later reuse.
- **Funding:** Acquisition of financial support for the trial leading to this publication.
- **Project administration:** Management, coordination, planning, and execution of trial.
- **Supervision:** Oversight and leadership responsibility for the research activity planning and execution, including mentorship external to the core team.

Suggested trial-specific roles not included in CRediT:
- **Site principal investigator:** The trialist or principal investigator responsible for coordinating all trial affairs at a participating center.
- **Statistical analysis plan:** Development of the analysis outlined in the trial registration and protocol into a detailed, *a priori* statistical analysis plan of the primary outcome, secondary outcomes, and other variables, before the dataset is closed and prepared for formal analysis.
- **Patient and public involvement:** Contribution from lay members of the public in areas such as trial priority setting, core outcome selection, proposal development, participant recruitment and retention.

CRediT roles rarely reported in published trials:
- **Resources:** Provision of study materials, computing resources, etc.
- **Software:** Programming, software development, designing computer programs, implementation of the computer code and supporting algorithms, etc.
- **Validation:** Replication or reproducibility of results.
- **Visualization:** Preparation of data presentation.

Source: DOI's:10.1087/20150211; 10.21037/atm.2019.12.96.

Unethical authorship

Authorship traditions vary across different fields and disciplines of health research. In trials, there is a tendency toward a higher number of authors per article due to the multidisciplinary and collaborative nature of the work, especially in multicenter trials. Theoretically, there may exist explicit definitions of authorship and contributions (Boxes 8.1 and 8.2). However, the practical operationalization of these is determined by disciplinary culture and institutional subcultures. Subjective interpretation is the norm in the application of authorship criteria. Authorship criteria serve to protect the status of authorship for those who have made contributions, but human nature, coupled with the pressure to publish or perish, can lead those in positions of power to impose their co-authorship on work without contributing. They can also prevent others from qualifying as authors, for example, by denying them the opportunity to meet the criteria related to drafting the work and its final approval (Box 8.1). Various forms of authorship abuse exist in the clinical research ecosystem (Box 8.3).

In multi-country trials, participating centers from less developed countries often randomize and follow up many participants. The data thus obtained meets the ICMJE data acquisition criterion for authorship. However, their developed country partners may exclude them from taking part in drafting the manuscript and its final approval, thus excluding them from authorship. This experience may be linked to perceptions of lower competence among developing country partners by researchers from developed countries. This perception may be compounded by stereotypes such as English language incompetence. Such biases even exist in developed countries where the native language is not English. The global code of conduct for equitable research partnerships stipulates the inclusion of developing country partners in the authorship of publications. The responsibility for defining who qualifies as an author and what their individual contributions are should ideally involve all those who participated in the trial. Institutions should ensure that all those and only those who make substantial contributions are included in the authorship list. However, the general observation is that institutional policies that promote unhealthy competition, such as "publish or perish", tend to undermine authorship integrity. In recent decades, there has also been a rise in authorship with multiple institutional affiliations. It would be wise to limit the affiliation listing to institutions where the trial actually took place.

Paper mills, a relatively recent phenomenon impinging strongly on responsible publication practices, have caught genuine publishers off guard (Chapter 7). Producing fake (plagiarized or fabricated) papers and selling authorship on them has become a global business. Legitimate publishers

Authorship abuse: Unethical authorship, including naming authors not strictly based on contribution, such as guest authorship, ghost authorship, invented authorship, and more (Box 8.3).

Committee on Publication Ethics (COPE): Issues guidance to journals on handling authorship disputes (publicationethics.org).

Ethics dumping: Exploitative practices that take advantage of the imbalance of power in research partnerships between high-income and lower-income settings.

Power: The ability to influence others. The role asymmetry in a relationship permits the powerful to influence the vulnerable. The responsibility to prevent influence from turning into abuse lies with the powerful party.

Paper mills: The business of publishing fake research papers and selling authorship.

Box 8.3: Various forms of unethical authorship

Coercion authorship	Bullying the research team into accepting them as a guest author, usually exercised by individuals in positions of power.
Collaboration authorship	Individuals collaborating and conveniently including each other as co-authors on a series of papers without making substantial contribution to all the papers in the series.
Ghost authorship	Purposefully not listing as co-author someone who has made substantial contributions, e.g., to avoid revealing the industry that originated the trial, making it look like an academic investigator-led project. Conflict of interest mismanagement is research misconduct (Chapter 10).
Gift authorship	A form of guest co-authorship offered or sought in the context of mentorship or as a goodwill gesture in advance of future research collaboration.
Guest authorship	Listing individuals as co-authors who have not made substantial contributions. Synonyms for guest include courtesy, gift, and honorary.
Highly prolific authorship	Authors who publish one full paper every five days (more than 72 full papers annually) may be achieved without meeting authorship criteria.
Invented authorship	Naming a fictitious person or a colleague as co-author without their permission.
Orphan authorship	Exploiting a power imbalance to exclude someone as a co-author, such as trainees or colleagues who have left the institution. The gender gap and low representation of contributors from less developed countries may be due to power imbalances.
Paid authorship	Buying co-authorship without making a contribution in a genuine or a fake paper (see Chapter 7 for paper mills).

This is not a complete list. For details of the terminology, see relevant sections in the text and the glossary.

have now picked up this issue and are beginning to identify and retract papers with paid authorship. Paid authorship is not necessarily linked to fake papers. Authorship can also be bought or sold on genuine papers. One sign that this might be happening is that authorship additions are requested while the paper is under journal's assessment and close to being accepted. Changes requested to authorship after submission are viewed with extreme concern. If honest trialists need to do this for a genuine reason, there is a good chance that a lot of explanation will be required to convince the journal editors.

Authorship in multicenter trials

How should trialists deal with the vexed issue of authorship? For single-center trials with few contributors who know each other well and have a history of working collaboratively, this may be easily settled without dispute. However, the trend is moving towards multicenter trials, because they offer the real possibility of delivering robust, useful evidence. In multicenter trials, however, authorship would not be quite straightforward. The proverb "success has many fathers, but failure is an orphan" is apt for successfully completed multicenter trials. Working in small groups is often a recipe for failed trials. To achieve large target sample sizes in a timely fashion, there is no option but to seek the help of many, even those previously unknown to original trialists, such as those from other countries and continents who do not even speak the same language, may be invited to take part. On the one hand, without collaboration, multicenter trials are unfeasible; on the other, the criteria for authorship are unsuitable for the types of collaborations these trials demand. Ideally, collaboration and co-authorship should go hand in hand, ensuring that colleagues in the centers where the trial is conducted, i.e., where recruitment takes place and outcome data are collected, are given credit. A related issue is determining the number of authors to be named from each center and the order of their authorship.

The issue of authorship in trials can be further complicated by the fact that individuals who make substantial contributions may join along the way after the trial has been designed and initiated, for example, to rescue a trial that is failing to recruit. Similarly, those who originally designed the trial and published its protocol may withdraw during the course, due to moving jobs or retiring, for instance. Thus, the initially conceived authorship may need modifications as the trial progresses towards completion. The solution to the authorship problem lies in forward planning. Ideally, each co-author should be able to identify the roles of other co-authors and have confidence in the integrity of their contributions. In large multicenter trials, with the best will in the world, this may prove difficult to achieve. There is no magic formula that would work in all types of situations. Each trial has its own unique character. Mutual discussion and documentation among those involved offer the most reasonable way forward to reach an agreement when submitting the manuscript. It is considered better to take a liberal approach in the interpretation of ICMJE authorship criteria, in the spirit of collaboration. As well as preventing authorship disputes and misconduct allegations post-publication, this approach will help deliver useful evidence for evidence-based medicine.

Authorship discussions could be started even before the trial starts recruitment. Theoretically, all members of the group named as authors

Usefulness of trials: A multidimensional concept, evaluating integrity, research priority, pragmatism, validity, precision, and more.

Site principal investigator: The trialist or investigator coordinating all trial affairs in a trial site or center. Since there can be no trial without randomized participants who have complete follow-up data, this role is recognized in trial authorship or acknowledgment.

Clinical investigator: Healthcare professionals who execute trials in clinical practice according to the approved protocol. When a trial site has many clinical investigators, one of them serves as the site principal investigator.

should meet all the four ICMJE authorship criteria (Box 8.1). They are also be expected as individuals to formally complete authorship statements and disclosure forms. In some large multi-author trials, authorship may be designated by a group name, with the names of individual members provided elsewhere in the manuscript. The individual authors are listed within the group name in bibliographic databases such as PubMed. The group name may be accompanied by names of some individual authors who may have taken a greater part in the trial than the rest of the trial team, and therefore wish to take greater credit. Such hybrids may appear as "authors and research group" or "authors on behalf of research group". It is the collective responsibility of the authors to settle the authorship format. Journals tend to stay out of arbitrating over who qualifies or does not qualify for authorship, what is the most suitable authorship format, the right authorship order, and more. With respect to group authorship, journals should be particular about the matter of responsibility for the integrity of the trial. The alphabetical order of listing authors is uncommon in health research. Sometimes, for site investigators, the authorship order is based on the number of participants randomized or the proportion of complete follow-ups, giving greater credit to sites that contributed more participants and outcome data. This helps meet the data acquisition criterion for authorship. These criteria should be considered very carefully, as they may inadvertently introduce a form of measurement bias. For example, if site principal investigators or clinical investigators target these criteria for improving their ranking in authorship, they may become the subject of manipulation. If agreement on authorship cannot be reached, the institutions where the work took place, not the journal, should be asked to adjudicate. This, of course, has the potential to open a Pandora's box when competing institutions attempt to collaborate. Institutional partnership agreements may be established to help address these issues.

Typically, institutions do not centrally handle authorship disputes as they do with investigations of research misconduct allegations (Chapter 10). Instead, this matter is delegated locally to the researchers who undertook the trial to sort it out among themselves. The corresponding author, the chief investigator, and trial management groups have the responsibility in this regard. If they cannot settle the matter, then the local departmental or divisional administration in charge of the trialists is expected to resolve it. Failing this, the institute's central administration may be approached to help settle the dispute. Disgruntled authors may even approach the courts to seek a legal resolution. If authors request the removal or addition of an author or the change of authorship order post-submission or post-publication, journals would likely seek signed statements of agreement from all the originally and finally listed authors for the requested change (see paper mills and unethical authorship above).

Chief investigator: The trialist, in some academic cultures also known as principal investigator, who is responsible for the conduct of the whole trial throughout its lifecycle from inception to publication. The chief investigator heads the trial management group and may appear as the first, last, or corresponding author of the trial on its publication.

Trial management group: Comprising of co-investigators and appointed trial staff, it is led by the chief investigator to oversee the conduct of the trial.

Box 8.4: Issues and considerations in authorship of trials

Factors	Issues	Methods	Considerations
Useful evidence is based on sizable, statistically powerful trials requiring many centers and a large number of contributors.	• Naming the first, last and corresponding authors • Constructing the order of authorship • Group vs. byline (individually named) authorship • Hybrid individual plus group authorship	• Informal consensus • Formal consensus • Scoring systems • Self-assessment • Peer-assessment • Hybrid • Authorship contract • Publication committee	• The ICMJE criteria are too rigid for trials. • Successful trials need many co-authors, including site principal investigators and patient representatives.

Source: DOI: 10.1111/j.1399-6576.2011.02477.x.

One way to proactively address the authorship issue is to enter into a formal authorship agreement or contract at an early stage of the trial, ideally before the first participant is randomized. In multicenter trials, it would not be a bad idea to establish a publication committee that can examine and document authorship issues as the trial progresses, along with planning the write-up. For example, the committee may seek 1–2 or more trialists from each participating center as co-authors depending on center's size and contribution, or it may determine a threshold based on the number of participants randomized as an internal criterion for authorship. There may be more than one paper planned, and requests may be made for sub-studies by the participating centers. Each of these various outputs will need to address authorship issues. Box 8.4 outlines the factors to explicitly consider in respect of authorship planning.

Acknowledgments

In a published paper, this section is usually placed somewhere between the end of the main text and the references. Non-author contributors should be named in acknowledgments. These contributions may be identified using the roles described above in Boxes 8.1 and 8.2.

The names of independent members of the data monitoring committee and the trial steering committee should be noted here, not in authorship (Chapter 6). The same applies to independent members of committees for adjudication of outcomes and adverse events. For undertaking trial activities related to its oversight, there should be no expectation from the outset to be named as authors, although trialists should not be surprised by the level of ignorance on this issue. There should be

Data Monitoring Committee (DMC), composed of independent experts, reports to the Trial Steering Committee (TSC) and makes recommendations regarding trial continuation, modification, or termination. The TSC, composed of an independent chair, members, and some of the trialists, is responsible for overall trial supervision and its chair gives instructions to the trial management group.

complete clarity on this matter. The names of these independent trial oversight committee members cannot be included in authorship; otherwise, how could they remain independent? Because acknowledgment may imply endorsement of the trial, journals may require written permission from the named individuals.

The question of how the scientific use of generative Artificial Intelligence (AI) should be honestly and transparently handled is hotly debated. AI, a subject within the computer science discipline, has developed large language models. These models have the capacity to respond to a scientific query automatically, using thousands of resources from the Internet without intellectual input from the scientist. Generative Pre-trained Transformer (ChatGPT) is one example of such an AI tool. It can be used in manuscript writing, peer review, and editing amongst many other possibilities in the publishing process. It has appeared in authorship of some scientific articles. It has been argued that authorship is accompanied by moral responsibility, something that only humans can provide. Thus, generative AI cannot be credited with authorship. Regarding its use in scientific articles, honest and transparent disclosure is required. Current recommendations state that its use should be acknowledged. If professional medical writing input has been sought in preparing the trial manuscript, its contribution should be acknowledged. Guidance exists on responsible publication when using professional manuscript writing services.

Citizens as co-authors

Paternalistic medicine is, or should be, a thing of the past. Patients are no longer just passive participants randomized and followed up as subjects in trials (Chapter 5). In recent years, there has been growing awareness of the importance of including the perspectives of citizens, patients, and carers in research design, particularly in setting priorities for trials, selection of core outcomes, development of protocols including consent procedures and patient information, planning recruitment and retention of participants, and dissemination of findings. This way the input of lay members of the public, in their capacity as family members, carers, and patients with lived experience of disease, helps improve the relevance, design, conduct, and reporting of trials. Lay representatives may also serve as independent members of trial steering committees.

In light of the above, citizens as patient representatives have a recognized role in trials, and the role they play should be recognized in authorship or acknowledgment, not brushed under the proverbial carpet. The ICMJE authorship criteria and CRediT are both unsuitable for dealing with this proposition as citizens' consultative roles go unrecognized in their

---

Good Publication Practice (GPP): Guidance in professional medical writing (DOI: 10.7326/M15-0288).

ChatGPT: A generative AI tool that may be deployed to draft and revise manuscripts among other scientific tasks. Its role should be recognized in the acknowledgment, not in trial authorship.

Citizen science: An open science initiative encouraging public and consumer involvement in scientific research with citizens actively making intellectual contributions.

Guidance for Reporting Involvement of Patients and the Public (GRIPP): Guidance for reporting citizen involvement in research (DOI: 10.1136/bmj.j3453).

Authors and Consumers Together Impacting on eVidencE (ACTIVE): A framework for citizen involvement in evidence syntheses, DOI: 10.1177/1355819619841647.

guidance at the time of writing this book. A greater contribution merits authorship, and a lesser contribution points toward acknowledgment. Reporting checklists for describing patient, carer, and public involvement in research exist, such as GRIPP, and ACTIVE. The guidance they offer may also help trialists learn how best to quantify the contribution of citizens towards authorship or acknowledgment in publications of trials.

Chapter 8: Authorship of trials – Key Points

Execution of trials (advice to trialists):

- Start discussions about authorship early, even before you start enrolling participants. Agree on authorship order mutually. A publication committee may be established to deal with this issue, depending on the number of trialists and centers involved.
- Engage patients, carers, and public representatives involved in trial co-production early with a view to inviting them to join the trial as co-authors.
- Report contributions transparently (see writing tips below). An explicit format like the one outlined in Box 8.2 offers a good starting point for descriptions of roles.
- If an authorship dispute arises, seek to settle the matter with institutional input before submitting the manuscript to the journal.
- The corresponding author or another delegated co-author must ensure completion of all the journal's administrative requirements, such as providing details of authorship, human research ethics committee approvals, trial registration documentation, protocol, statistical analysis plan, funding disclosures, declarations of conflicts of interests, etc. Retain signed authorship agreements and related declarations even if the journal does not seek such documents. The corresponding author should be available throughout the submission, peer review, and post-publication process to respond in a timely manner.
- If the journal does not automatically share information with all authors, the corresponding author should send copies of all correspondence with journals to all co-authors.
- Never use a paper mill. Never buy or sell authorship (Chapter 7).

Conflicts of interest: A potential or perceived compromise in the objectivity or judgment of anyone involved in research and publication due to financial or personal (non-financial) interests. Failure to declare is considered research misconduct.

Writing tips for trial authors

- **Title page:** List authorship in the format and order agreed with the contributors, and in a format acceptable to the journal. If group authorship is used, state clearly where the group members can be found, for example, in the acknowledgment section, in a table in the main text, or in the supplementary material. Ensure that equal credit for first or last author positions in the authorship order is clearly mentioned, if required. Use unique digital author identifiers, such as ORCID, for all those named. Limit the institutional affiliation listing to those where the trial actually took place.
- **Methods:** Patient, carer, and public involvement may be described here with or without the naming of citizens involved in trial co-production, depending on the journal's instructions.
- **Tables:** It may be that the journal will ask you to include names of individuals in group authorship on the title page or in the acknowledgment section, but be imaginative and use other alternatives that suit your purpose better, such as a table in the manuscript may be deployed using roles included in Box 8.2. Give a detailed title that permits the table to stand alone.
- **Acknowledgments:** Name non-author contributors with their permission. Name independent members of trial oversight committees here or in the methods section depending on the journal's instructions. Acknowledge the use of generative AI.
- **Supplementary material:** Detailed contributions of all named in authorship and acknowledgment may be provided as a supplementary table using roles included in Box 8.2. Signed agreements for authorship and acknowledgments may be appended.

Roles of institutions, journals, and funders

- Institutions and funders should replace traditional metrics based on citation counts with those that value usefulness for society (Box 2.5), removing the pressure to publish or perish.
- Institutional incentives should recognize contributions (both authorship and acknowledgments) for appointments, annual appraisals, and promotions, and discourage authorship abuse.
- Institutions, journals, and funders should promote the recognition of patient, carer, and public involvement in authorship and acknowledgment.
- Journals should seek signed declarations of all those named in authorship and acknowledgment. The declaration should cover at least that the named authors fulfill authorship criteria, that

no individuals deserving of authorship have been omitted, and that authors accept responsibility for trial integrity. They should seek and publish contributor role descriptions for each author and those named in acknowledgments. Journals should be vigilant about the exclusion of contributors from developing countries in multi-country trials.

- Journals should correspond with all named co-authors in case someone has been included without their knowledge or permission.

- Journals and institutions should cooperate in timely investigations and correction of the research record where allegations of authorship abuse are made or if such abuse is suspected (Chapter 10).

- Funders should prioritize research on the evaluation of authorship characteristics (e.g., small number of trial authors relative to trial size, use of non-institutional email addresses, etc.; Box 7.4) as screening tests for trial integrity.

9 Evidence syntheses of randomized clinical trials

Evidence-based medicine: The conscientious, explicit, and judicious use of current best research evidence in making healthcare decisions. It ranks randomized clinical trials and their evidence syntheses at the top of the effectiveness evidence hierarchy.

Evidence syntheses of randomized clinical trials compile the highest level of evidence for informing clinical practice and policy. In addition to their own transparency, their trustworthiness depends on the integrity of the collated trials. So far, trial integrity assessment has not been incorporated within the evidence synthesis methodology. It is well-known that the editorial and peer review system established by journals are not true custodians of published trial integrity. Thus, the acquisition, assessment, and analysis of trials in reviews should be mindful of failures of responsible research conduct. Integrity assessments should become a routine part of evidence synthesis. Useful evidence syntheses are those that cover broader, not narrow, questions, as such reviews help both in planning new trials and in generating guidance for practice and policy. This chapter provides guidance on planning and conducting evidence syntheses of trials with explicit consideration given to the possibility that the literature available for review is polluted by trials with integrity flaws.

Evidence synthesis: A general term describing a systematic approach to collating evidence.

Trials and evidence syntheses

Systematic review: Summarizing the evidence using systematic and explicit methods to identify, select, and appraise relevant primary studies, and to extract, synthesize, and report their findings. Throughout this chapter, the term "review" refers to systematic review.

Trials and evidence syntheses go hand in hand. Have a look at the case study in Box 9.1. Trial protocols are prepared for human research ethics committee evaluation, including a justification of the trial priority. The trial itself needs a scientific justification. Both of these pillars of a trial's ethical justification are best constructed on the foundation of evidence synthesis (Chapter 4). During the course of the trial, reviewing the accumulating external evidence is an essential requirement for trial oversight (Chapter 6). The trial may be continued as planned, modified, or stopped early depending in part on the findings of the published external evidence synthesized. The publication of the trial findings should include a comparison with other studies. Ideally, the new trial findings should be used to update existing evidence syntheses. With data sharing becoming a standard requirement for responsible trial publication, evidence syntheses should benefit from Individual Participant Data (IPD) meta-analyses. To make trials useful in the context of real-world healthcare practice and policy, evidence syntheses, such as umbrella reviews, present an options appraisal addressing broad questions that compare the available interventions.

DOI: 10.1201/9781003461401-9

Box 9.1: Case study – Evidence syntheses published during a trial's lifecycle

- A trial published in 2009 started participant recruitment in 1998 after obtaining approvals.
- During the trial course, six evidence syntheses were published.
- A mapping review undertaken for trial protocol preparation was published in 1997.
- Two systematic reviews with meta-analysis were published in 2000 and 2005 during trial participant recruitment. Such evidence syntheses help in the deliberations related to trial oversight.
- A third systematic review with meta-analysis was published in 2007 during trial participant follow-up.
- A fourth systematic review with Individual Patient Data (IPD) meta-analysis was published in 2010, after trial publication, sharing its raw data with that shared by other trialists.
- The 2009 trial and the 2010 IPD meta-analysis demonstrated that the intervention was ineffective.
- An umbrella review, published in 2011–12, overviewed 35 systematic reviews covering the available options.

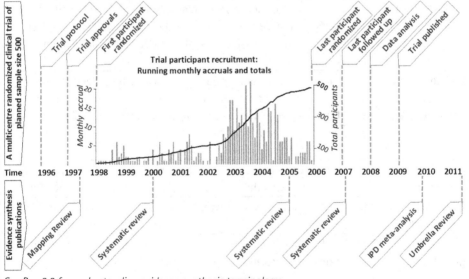

See Box 9.2 for understanding evidence synthesis terminology.
See Box 6.2 for the trial lifecycle.
Source: DOI's: 10.1001/jama.2009.1268;   10.1046/j.1365-2508.1999.00269.x;   10.1002/14651858.
CD001896;   10.1002/14651858.CD001896.pub2;   10.1080/00016340600753117;   10.1093/humupd/
dmq031; 10.1136/bmj.e3011.

Box 9.2: Understanding evidence synthesis nomenclature

Evidence synthesis	A general term describing a systematic approach to collating relevant evidence to address a research question, map the literature, create clinical practice guidelines, and more. The term "systematic review" is sometimes used synonymously.
Mapping review (scoping review)	An evidence synthesis of an exploratory nature undertaken to describe or map a wider research topic. Such evidence syntheses are called "scoping reviews" when the purpose is to clarify key concepts. These reviews are helpful in identifying gaps in the literature.
Systematic review	An evidence synthesis undertaken to address a research question. For example, a narrowly framed question may determine the effect of a single intervention (two-arm comparison) or a broad question may determine the effects of multiple interventions for the same disease or condition. Systematic reviews use explicit methods to identify, select, and appraise relevant trials, and to extract, collate, and report their findings. They may or may not use meta-analysis.
Meta-analysis	A statistical technique for combining (pooling) the reported results of multiple trials addressing the same question to produce a summary result. Trials are usually weighted according to some measure of their precision, such as the inverse of variance.
Individual Participant Data (IPD) meta-analysis	A meta-analysis that uses participant-level data collected in the included trials to produce a summary result. Data sharing makes IPD meta-analysis possible. This approach offers more statistically powerful analyses and is particularly useful in addressing secondary questions not prioritized in individual trials.
Umbrella review (overview)	A review of systematic reviews. Both narrow and broad questions can be addressed through umbrella reviews or systematic reviews.
Network meta-analysis	A meta-analytic technique that compares multiple interventions for the same condition using both direct and indirect evidence.
Clinical practice guideline	A collection of statements to assist practitioners and patients in making decisions about specific clinical situations. They often, but not always, use evidence syntheses.

Adapted from: DOI: 10.1201/9781003220039.
For details on the terminology used in evidence syntheses see relevant sections in the text, and the Glossary.

Outline of a systematic review

Evidence syntheses are ubiquitous. Around 1,000 systematic reviews are published weekly in the PubMed database alone. Boxes 9.2 and 9.3 outline the various evidence synthesis terms and methods. Systematic reviews of randomized clinical trials are a key tool in evidence-based medicine. They allow the best evidence to reach patients through clinical practice guidelines. To provide market access to newly approved drugs and devices, policymakers use them too. Systematic reviews also serve as standard background information in any trial protocol and both funders and human research ethics committees look closely at the findings of evidence syntheses to determine if a new trial would be scientifically justified. On trial completion, trialists often update systematic reviews with their new trial results to put their findings in the context of the existing trials. Throughout this chapter, the term "review" refers to systematic reviews.

Briefly covering the standard review methodology, the first step involves framing structured questions using the same approach outlined in Box 2.1. The problem to be addressed should be specified clearly and unambiguously, defining the participants, interventions, and outcomes. The review question may be narrow or broad. The latter permits reviews to be more useful in getting trial evidence into practice. The second step involves conducting searches to identify the relevant trials. An extensive search typically interrogates multiple databases without time and language restrictions. Journals' bias in favor of publishing positive findings requires that the literature searches are conducted with the intent to reduce the risk of missing out on trials with negative results. The selection criteria, which follow directly from the review question, are used to short-list citations for full-text assessment. The reasons for the exclusion of full texts are recorded in an appendix to accompany the published systematic review article. The third step assesses the quality of the trials included, examining the risk of bias in depth, looking at features outlined in Box 2.2. These detailed quality assessments help in several ways, such as exploring quality variation as the reason for the heterogeneity of effects from trial to trial, and in informing decisions about undertaking statistical syntheses.

The fourth step summarizes the evidence and data using tables and graphs. Statistical methods may be deployed to examine the differences between trial effects. Too much heterogeneity may preclude meta-analysis. On the other hand, the appropriate use of meta-analysis may combine individual trial effects to help produce more precise overall results, such as narrower confidence intervals (Box 2.4). This approach may allow the combination of several small explanatory trials which individually may be useless on account of their imprecise results. Metaphorically, if this works, a meta-analysis could be said to be capable of turning noise into a signal. The fifth and final step interprets the findings judiciously, considering the

Clinical practice guideline: Statements that aim to assist practitioners and patients in making decisions about specific clinical situations.

Effect: The statistic capturing the observed association between interventions and outcomes. It has a point estimate and a confidence interval.

Meta-analysis: A statistical technique for combining (pooling) the results of multiple trials addressing the same question to produce a summary result.

Heterogeneity: The degree to which the individual trial effects in a systematic review are similar or different.

Publication bias: The likelihood of publication of a trial is related to the significance of its results. Funnel plots explore the risk of publication and related biases.

Box 9.3: Some terms and methods applied in evidence synthesis of randomized clinical trials

Study quality assessment	Assessment of the degree to which a trial included in an evidence synthesis has minimized the risk of various biases, focusing on trial validity (internal) (Box 2.2). Bias assessment is distinct from integrity assessment.
Integrity assessment	Assessment of the risk that a trial included in an evidence synthesis has integrity flaws or it harbors irresponsible research conduct (Box 7.4). Integrity assessment is distinct from study quality (risk of bias) assessment.
Funnel plot	A scatter plot of individual trial effects included in a systematic review against a measure of trial precision, such as trial size, or inverse of variance. Funnel asymmetry is examined to look for publication and related biases.
Forest plot	A graphical display of individual trial effects (with 95% confidence intervals) included in a systematic review addressing a narrow question (two-arm comparison), along with the summary effect if meta-analysis is applied (Box 2.4).
Subgroup analysis	Meta-analyses conducted in subgroups of trials stratified by differences in various trial characteristics (Box 9.4).
Meta-regression	A multivariable model with individual trial effects as dependent variables and various trial characteristics as independent variables. Trials are usually weighted according to some measure of their precision, such as inverse of variance.
Treatment network	A diagrammatic presentation of the interventions covered in a systematic review or umbrella review addressing a broad question evaluating multiple treatment options for the same disease or condition. It gives a bird's-eye view of all the interventions that exist, the ones that have been directly compared (two-arm comparisons) and which can be compared indirectly.
Evidence strength	The extent to which there can be confidence that the summary effect estimate in an evidence synthesis is correct. Integrity flaws, heterogeneity, imprecision, risk of bias, funnel asymmetry, etc. downgrade evidence strength.

Source: DOI: 10.1201/9781003220039.
For details on the terminology used and the proposed methods for incorporating integrity assessment in evidence syntheses see Box 9.5, relevant section in the text, and the Glossary.

output of the various analyses. For example, poor quality (high risk of bias), heterogeneity (conflicting results with both positive and negative findings), imprecision (results with wide confidence intervals), and risk of publication bias may downgrade the strength of the evidence. Thus, the recommendations generated for practice may be weak, although such a review could provide a strong justification for launching a new trial.

Trial integrity and evidence syntheses

Even though today's trials obtain ethics approval, register prospectively, and apply oversight during trial conduct, they are by no means foolproof. There is always the possibility of unintentional errors, carelessness, flawed protocol implementation, and other issues that can lead to integrity deviations. Thus, there are trials with integrity flaws in the literature pool available to reviewers. Systematic review methods have to routinely deploy trial integrity assessments. There are published trials with retractions, corrigenda, and expressions of concerns issued by journals. These notices probably represent the tip of the iceberg. Allegations are made by data sleuths via blogging and social media, including academic online platforms such as PubPeer (pubpeer.com) and Retraction Watch (retractionwatch.com). It is well-recognized that the journal mechanism for the correction of erroneous and fraudulent literature is flawed. There is probably also a pool of trials whose integrity has never been questioned, but they may harbor integrity flaws (Box 3.1). Defective trials should never enter the scientific record, but they do and once there they are hard to remove. The close cooperation required between institutions and journals for effective, timely research record correction, is lacking. The problem evidence synthesis faces is highlighted with a case study in Box 9.4.

Until recently, review methodology has not explicitly targeted trial integrity. However, it is now recognized that reviewers' reliance on the assessment system established by journals as the custodian of research integrity was either poor judgment or blind faith. In the past, only a small proportion of evidence syntheses have been corrected or retracted on the discovery of proven integrity flaws among their included trials (see examples in Boxes 2.4 and 9.4). There is now a realization that the issue of included trial integrity failures cannot be brushed under the carpet. Without a formal assessment of responsible research conduct among trials being considered for inclusion in evidence syntheses, there is a possibility that those without integrity may slip in alongside genuine data. This is a particular concern because the meta-analytic summary estimates of the overall effect are modestly sensitive to the presence of flawed data (DOI: 10.1080/08989621.2021.1947810). Such statistical summaries may lead to erroneous inferences. If these findings go forward unchecked into

Data sleuthing: Post-publication investigation of possible research misconduct and questionable research practices by volunteer researchers.

Research integrity: Undertaking trials in accordance with ethical and professional principles and standards. Integrity failures may result from honest errors or deliberate misconduct. Responsible research conduct paves the way for trial methods and findings to be regarded as trustworthy.

Retraction: The removal of a published paper from the research record due to, for example, the discovery of a flaw in its integrity.

Expression of concern: A note published by a journal to inform readers of a potential concern regarding the integrity of a paper.

Box 9.4: Case study – Meta-analysis retracted and republished

- During the COVID-19 pandemic, ivermectin, an antiparasitic drug, was considered a possible treatment.
- In July 2021, a published meta-analysis suggested an improvement in outcomes with ivermectin.
- The same month, an included trial was retracted.
- In August 2021, an expression of concern was issued by the journal about the meta-analysis.
- In October 2021, another included trial was retracted.
- The original meta-analysis was retracted by the journal.
- In January 2022, the journal republished a revised meta-analysis. The overall meta-analytic findings were not emphasized. The subgroup meta-analysis showed that the effect on outcome was underpinned by the retracted and the poor-quality trials. In the subgroup of good-quality trials, there was no effect.

Source: DOI's: 10.3390/v13112154; 10.21203/rs.3.rs-100956/v2; 10.1093/ofid/ofab645.

---

clinical practice guidelines, the recommendations made for healthcare practice may be erroneous too. Thus, a revamp of the evidence synthesis methodology is needed.

Incorporating trial integrity assessment in systematic reviews

Box 9.5 outlines the explicit consideration of trial integrity assessment at each step of a systematic review. An evidence synthesis, mindful of research integrity, should clarify upfront the focus on trustworthy trials when framing its question. It must use explicit methods to detect citations with integrity concerns, excluding trials with proven integrity flaws covered in retraction notices, corrigenda, expressions of concerns, letters to editors, and public comments on platforms such as PubPeer. Specific searches should be undertaken for retractions, such as in the Retraction Watch database (retractiondatabase.org), or through the use of specific search filters for capturing such citations in general bibliographic databases. Data extraction should target transparency features, such as prospective registration, conflicts of interest, funding sources, data sharing statements, missing data, and more. The integrity assessment is distinct from the trial quality (risk of bias) assessment. For example, too much missing data relates to bias, whereas too little missing data relate to integrity. Selective outcome reporting is another example. At first glance, it may seem like a bias-related feature, but the possibility of p-hacking

Selective outcome reporting: A difference in the outcomes reported in a published trial compared to its protocol and prospective registration.

Sensitivity analysis: Repetition of an analysis under different assumptions to examine the impact of these assumptions on the results.

would turn it into an integrity flaw (Chapter 5). This is because if different statistical tests have been repeated until one shows significance, i.e., p-value < 0.05, then data analysis has been manipulated. The trial statistical analysis plan would need to be examined for the delineation of a single pre-specified primary analysis (Box 5.2). Data tabulation should routinely include descriptions of integrity features when describing trial characteristics. Heterogeneity assessments including inspection of forest plots and funnel plots should look for outliers against predefined thresholds for implausibly extreme effects. This is important as extreme effects may arise due to chance in small trustworthy trials. The outlier analysis may be used to exclude trials, or to perform sensitivity analyses. In statistical syntheses, integrity-based meta-regression and subgroup analyses should be planned. Inferences should downgrade evidence with integrity concerns when generating recommendations.

A key aspect of the methodology outlined above is determining how to proceed after excluding retracted trials with proven misconduct. What to do when trials have some publicly expressed concerns or issues identified during integrity assessment, but without any proven misconduct? This is not a new controversy when viewed in historical terms. In the earlier days of reviewing effectiveness evidence, observational studies where investigators did not attempt to create the group allocation, were excluded. However, studies allocating participants to groups using open, totally predictable assignment methods, such as according to birth dates, and odd-even alternation, were included along with genuinely randomized trials. They were even given a specific name, "quasi-randomized studies", to raise their level of merit above cohort studies, even though they suffered all the same methodological biases that were inherent in the observational design. Fast forward to the current day, quasi-randomized studies are excluded from consideration altogether. This is analogous to the current situation, where integrity-conscious reviews might decide to include trials based on a research transparency feature, such as prospective registration. Trials without prospective registration will then be removed from consideration altogether in the evidence synthesis. History repeats itself. Pseudo-randomized trials and those not prospectively registered might become part of the same bin of history. As evidence syntheses begin to incorporate integrity assessments, reviewers do not have to look for reports of whether or not misconduct is proven. If they have validated instruments or markers providing proxies for integrity concerns, they can simply construct them as part of the exclusion criteria.

Forest plot: A graphical display of individual trial effects with 95% confidence intervals in a systematic review alongside the meta-analytic summary effect.

Transparency in research: Open research practices, including prospective registration, adherence to trial design, *a priori* statistical analysis plan, data sharing, and timely and complete public reporting.

Box 9.5: Steps of evidence syntheses incorporating trial integrity assessments

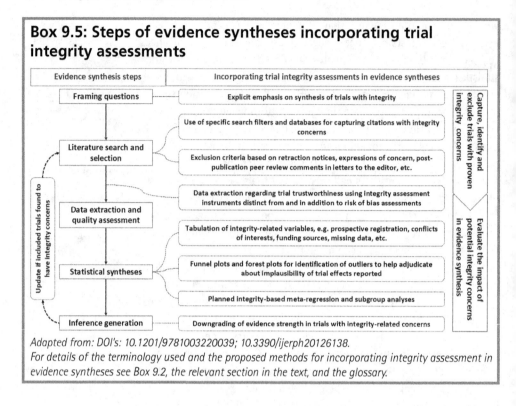

Adapted from: DOI's: 10.1201/9781003220039; 10.3390/ijerph20126138.
For details of the terminology used and the proposed methods for incorporating integrity assessment in evidence syntheses see Box 9.2, the relevant section in the text, and the glossary.

Those studies that pass the integrity-related inclusion criteria may still have some integrity concerns. For example, trials with prospective registration may have evidence of selective outcome reporting with p-hacking (Chapter 5). Thus, in addition to using an integrity feature as a basic trial selection criterion, there is a need to perform a more detailed integrity assessment of the selected trials. The differences between the prospectively registered trial and that reported in the published trial may be based on changes to the protocol of the ongoing trial advised by independent trial supervisors, or it may be the result of p-hacking. Various versions of the trial protocol since its original approval, its *a priori* statistical analysis plan prepared ahead of the dataset closure, conference abstracts or posters of the trial presented before its publication in a journal, and other related documents could shed light on this matter. It is important to distinguish the difference between planned protocol changes and trickery, and adjust the detailed integrity assessment accordingly. Historically, this aspect is the same as the inclusion of trials that are genuinely randomized, but have varying levels of risk of bias, such as those arising due to faulty allocation concealment, lack of blinding, etc. In earlier days of reviewing, no detailed quality (risk of bias) assessments were performed among the included tri-

Funnel plot: A scatter plot of individual trial effects in a systematic review against a measure of trial precision, such as the inverse of variance. Funnel asymmetry suggests the possibility of publication and related biases.

als. Today, it is inconceivable that a review could skip the step of risk of bias assessment and proceed directly to meta-analysis after trial selection. To get to today's level of advance in this area of methodology, items included in the risk of bias checklists have been validated through theoretical and empirical studies. The quality assessments are routinely used in planned meta-regression and subgroup analyses, as well as in grading the strength of evidence for generating inferences and recommendations for practice. The same approach should be deployed when developing and incorporating integrity assessments in evidence syntheses.

Developments required for trial integrity assessments in evidence syntheses

Just as this book covered critical appraisal of trials in Chapter 1, critical appraisal of evidence syntheses of trials is also an important feature. Reporting checklists for publishing evidence syntheses are many, such as PRISMA and MARS. There are also several instruments available for assessing the quality of systematic reviews, such as AMSTAR-2 and ROBIS, and clinical practice guidelines, such as RIGHT and AGREE II. These include items within domains that address how the evidence syntheses have acquired, appraised, and analyzed trial data. They cover trial quality assessment with respect to the risk of bias, but integrity assessments do not feature in their present versions. These checklists or instruments need updating to be fit-for-purpose in the new era of trial-integrity-conscious evidence synthesis.

Ongoing development of methods to help incorporate integrity assessments in evidence synthesis is needed. Search filters must be constructed to identify literature with integrity flaws and tested for performance, as such citations tend to be badly signposted. A unified platform bringing together retractions, corrigenda, and post-publication comments about trials with integrity concerns is required. The enormous literature size and growth of publication numbers is a related challenge, particularly when one considers the recent paper mills scandal, i.e., the production of totally fake papers. To accurately detect integrity breaches in publicly available trials, instrument validation research is required. The currently available integrity assessment instruments, apart from plagiarism or image integrity checks, are not based on empirical research. They have a theoretical basis and case studies demonstrating their use. What is needed is research formally establishing their performance (face, content, construct, and criterion validity). An important aspect is the assessment of ethics and consent standards in trials,

Subgroup analysis: Meta-analyses carried out in subgroups of trials stratified according to differences in trial features, such as trial integrity.

Instrument: A systematic approach to measurement for accurately quantifying and categorizing observations for attributing meaning. Checklists used for review quality assessment, such as AMSTAR, and ROBIS, are validated measurement instruments or tools.

Variance: A statistical measure of variation in terms of the deviations of individual observations from the mean value. The inverse of variance is often used to weight trials in statistical syntheses, e.g., meta-analysis, meta-regression, and funnel plot analysis. This weighting makes the individual trials with lower variance (i.e., with less random error or greater precision in estimation of trial effect) to have more importance in the calculations.

as the term "integrity" covers both ethical and professional principles and standards. It cannot be that data fraud detection is targeted for assessment, but breaches of basic human rights, such as those inherent in flawed consent procedures, are overlooked. Deficits in informed consent should feature in integrity assessments (Chapter 4). The precise characterization of research integrity distinct from quality (risk of bias) assessments is required. Avoiding confusion over the concepts of bias and integrity is key. Perhaps the term "quality" needs a new definition; it may include bias and integrity as two categories or constructs, each with its separate assessment. Time will tell how the terminology issue will be settled in the future.

Further developments are needed to better understand how the existing graphical and statistical methods applied in evidence syntheses can be used in addressing trial integrity. For example, the funnel plot methodology that exists for examining missing small studies could be redesigned to inspect small studies that have implausibly large effects. Similarly, the techniques for heterogeneity assessment embedded within forest plots could potentially be developed to look for outlier results. Exploration of reasons for heterogeneity with meta-regression can be readily adapted to include integrity assessments, as a dependent variable in the models. Subgroup analyses can prespecify integrity features as stratification variables (Box 9.4). With the introduction of multiple testing, there would be the need for managing the risk of spurious significance, e.g., with a more stringent statistical significance threshold (p-value < 0.01). Alongside this, the methodology for assessing the strength of the evidence collated in systematic reviews will need to incorporate integrity risk as a domain. Downgrading evidence this way will inevitably have a downstream impact on generating recommendations. Transparency in generating inferences will take center stage in creating clinical practice guidelines.

Data sharing in trials is expected to become the norm going forward. Meta-analyses will likely routinely be able to seek Individual Participant Data (IPD) with this development. How should one apply statistical techniques to detect anomalous patterns to check for data integrity? Could these techniques be applied to determine exclusion criteria? As things stand, reviews take too much time. Asking reviewers to do even more tasks, some of which will require new learning, does not sound fair. Beware that automation will continue to grow as computer sciences develop. This will help in many review aspects including integrity assessments via automated data extraction as well as graphical and statistical analyses. Periodic update policies in reviews should include integrity concerns (retraction, corrigendum, expression of concern) identified in included trials after review publication, and this will also be assisted by the use of artificial intelligence.

Meta-regression: A multivariable model with effects of individual trials (weighted according to a measure of precision, such as the inverse of variance) as the dependent variable and various trial characteristics, such as trial integrity and quality, as independent variables.

Individual Participant Data (IPD) meta-analysis: A meta-analysis that uses raw data collected in the included trials.

Artificial Intelligence (AI): Automated solutions using methods like machine learning, natural language processing, data mining, information retrieval, and other computer science methods.

Controversial aspects of integrity assessments in evidence syntheses

There are many controversial issues to consider. For a start: Would reviewers be expected to raise complaints when they identify integrity concerns? One view is that reviewers simply should be mindful of the risk of integrity flaws without the need to raise any doubts about the intellectual honesty of trialists, peer-reviewers, and editors. They should purely focus on undertaking their evidenced syntheses with integrity, leaving aside the issue of whistleblowing and research record correction. Their reviews should protect patients and public health from the risk posed by evidence pollution due to trial integrity failures, not stray into controversy outside their sphere.

Integrity assessment incorporated in reviews will serve as a form of post-publication peer review. If the original trial authors wish to remark on the review's integrity assessment, they will be able to use the letter to the editor section of the journal or other forums, such as PubPeer, to provide their responses publicly. The existing mechanisms in the research ecosystem should be strengthened to deal with the issues arising from integrity assessments in evidence syntheses. The reasons for failure to comply fully with responsible research conduct requirements in published trials include, among others, honest errors, lack of training, undeclared conflicts of interests, introduction of spin in the writeup, carelessness, recklessness, and deliberate fraud. It is not the reviewers' role to make judgments on these matters. Stakeholder organizations will need to define their roles in being alert to integrity concerns raised in evidence syntheses. The concerns should be investigated as research misconduct allegations (Chapter 10). Institutions, funders, journals, and other entities should have mechanisms in place to learn their own lessons for continuously strengthening their systems of governance and peer review. They will likely need to update their research integrity policies and procedures. All this effort should impact the research culture (Chapter 3).

Misconduct: Unethical or unprofessional research conduct that is intentional, reckless, or negligent. Honest error is not misconduct.

Questionable research practices: Irresponsible research practices that are regarded as unethical or unprofessional but fall short of being considered misconduct.

Institution: A clinical academic organization such as a university or a hospital, where trials take place. Institutions have primary responsibility for the ethical and professional conduct of their trials.

Journal: An establishment composed of editors and other publishing staff who organize peer review and publication of manuscripts of trials and their syntheses.

Usefulness of evidence syntheses of trials

Typically, randomized clinical trials address narrow questions focusing on the evaluation of a single intervention in a two-arm comparison (Chapter 2). Typical systematic reviews extend this two-arm comparison using meta-analyses to improve the precision of the effect, reducing the width of the confidence interval. This approach has merit, to an extent. However, the fundamental limitation of this approach is that real-world healthcare is not a two-arm comparison. The two-arm trial is fine when it comes to obtaining drug or device approval. However, this is not optimal when it comes to making real-world decisions. In the healthcare setting, i.e., in life as lived by patients and practitioners in the real world, there are many more than two options available for a particular disease or condition. Multi-arm trials are not common, being unfeasible on account of complexity, budgetary restrictions, and more. However, whenever several two-arm comparisons exist in trials, umbrella reviews or overviews collating all the systematic reviews of two-arm comparisons become feasible. They are particularly useful for creating clinical practice guidelines. Evidence syntheses should move towards the compilation of the comparative analyses of all available options for a disease or condition; this way they can become useful for informing healthcare practice and policy (Box 9.6).

The value given to pragmatism in trials can be extended to evidence syntheses to make them useful. To begin with, for incorporating research into practice, the appraisal of options should be broad-based, not narrow. Thus, the idea of framing review questions, including all interventions available here and now, is the first step in a fit-for-purpose evidence synthesis. The breadth of the question is what makes the synthesis useful. Umbrella reviews that collate several reviews on a narrow question fail at this first step. In such cases, umbrella review methodology serves to harmonize the interpretation across existing narrow systematic reviews, but it does not capture the real-world question. Umbrella reviews with broad questions, however, have the potential to underpin evidence-based medicine in real-world healthcare settings.

Having addressed the issue of question breadth, one can look at what can be gained by examining many interventions together. The first is the ability to have a bird's-eye overview of the evidence landscape. The variation of participant characteristics across trials can be examined. The interventions presented diagrammatically form what is called the treatment network (network meta-analysis derives its name from this). How many interventions exist, and which of these have been directly compared against each other (head-to-head comparisons), can be easily seen. It becomes possible to visualize the amount of evidence associated with each of the interventions. Then, it also becomes possible to see if interventions not directly compared, can be indirectly compared through a common comparator. For example, if A is compared with C and B is compared with C head-to-head, it becomes possible to compare A with B indirectly, using C as the common comparator. This approach can identify research gaps, pointing to an absence or scarcity of evidence for interventions. It can also help in the selection of a control group for comparison with trial intervention. This is part of the scientific justification of trials (Chapter 4).

Multi-arm multi-stage trial: A type of trial to assess multiple interventions with the option to continue, add, or discontinue trial arms at each interim statistical analysis according to a pre-specified plan. They aim to evaluate all available options for the treatment of a target disease or condition.

Pragmatism: The extent to which trials can be anticipated to produce useful results that directly inform healthcare practice and policy.

Usefulness of evidence syntheses: A multidimensional concept, evaluating integrity, research priority, pragmatism, validity, and precision.

Box 9.6: The usefulness of evidence syntheses of randomized clinical trials

Bed to bedside	Laboratory research	Early translation		Late translation			Use in practice
Study nomenclature		Safety, tolerability, dose finding, proof-of-concept	Explanatory or pilot trial	Confirmatory trial	Pragmatic trial		Surveillance
Research synthesis			Evidence syntheses of trials				
Evidence synthesis type			Systematic review		Umbrella review		
Integrity (trustworthiness) of evidence synthesis ----			Low transparency	—	High transparency		
Integrity (trustworthiness) of included trials --------			Low transparency	—	High transparency		
Societal priority of the review topic -------------			Low disease burden	—	High disease burden		
Participant characteristics ----------------			Narrow spectrum	—	Representative		
Comparison or control intervention ----------			Inactive or placebos	—	All options		
Number of options compared (arms) ---------			Few, two-arm	—	Multi-arm		
Outcomes ----------------------------			Patient-relevance low	—	Patient-relevant		
Statistical comparison ----------------			Direct only	—	Direct and indirect		
Statistical synthesis (meta-analysis) ---------			Pair-wise	—	Network		
Interpretation for practice and policy ---------			Low applicability	—	High applicability		

(Left axis: Pragmatism features; vertical middle: Less clinically useful → More clinically useful)

See: Box 1.2 for definitions of trial types; Box 9.1 for definitions of systematic and umbrella reviews. The demarcations between various stages and terms tend not to be as clear-cut as depicted; see glossary and text for explanations concerning the grey overlapping zones.
See Box 2.5 for the usefulness of randomized clinical trials.
Sources: DOI's: 10.1201/9781003220039; 10.1136/ebmed-2016-110599.

With dozens of options available and hundreds of trials within a topic, systematic reviews of two-arm comparisons fail to give the bird's eye overview. Multiple systematic reviews covering interventions for the same disease or condition create information overload. The human brain can only handle a finite amount of information at a given time, and when information is scattered, it becomes more difficult to manage it. There is a risk that viable options may be ignored in decision-making. For pragmatism, the comprehensive approach to compiling the evidence of all available options in one synthesis, and then comparing the options, directly and indirectly as feasible, is required. There are challenges and opportunities inherent in this approach. The statistical approach to data synthesis here, i.e., network meta-analysis, has its intricacies for review-ers to comprehend and master. It can generate a rank order of the available interventions, classifying them for their effectiveness. The steps in reviews covering search and selection, data extraction, and synthesis will all be more effortful in these comprehensive evidence syntheses. That said, as automation is developing, the human effort required in reviewing will likely change in its nature, providing supervision to machines performing the reviews. With integrity assessments incorporated in each one of the review steps, the prospect of truly useful evidence syntheses of trials is not far on the horizon.

Open science and evidence synthesis

Research integrity should be put center stage in the new era of evidence syntheses of trials. While performing integrity assessments of the trials included, reviewers should be mindful that charity begins at home. Their own work should meet the open science and transparency criteria. For example, prospective registration cannot just be a requirement for trials, it should be applied in evidence syntheses. Data sharing equally could not just be a requirement for trials, it should take place in reviews as well, so others can double-check and replicate the results reported. Funding disclosures and declarations of conflicts of interest should be standard in published evidence syntheses.

Research priority: The ranking or selection of a few among the many established research gaps and needs.

Research gap: A gap in knowledge.

Open science: An umbrella term covering various initiatives like open access publications, open peer review, open research data, and citizen science, that encourage sharing, cooperation, and knowledge dissemination without restrictions.

Chapter 9: Evidence syntheses of randomized clinical trials – Key points

Execution of evidence syntheses of trial (advice to trialists and reviewers)

- Plan evidence syntheses of trials for priority topics.
- Set trials in the context of existing evidence, undertaking evidence syntheses as part of trial planning (Chapters 4 and 5), conduct (Chapter 6), and completion (Chapter 7).
- Frame questions for reviews as broadly as possible, keeping in mind the usefulness of findings for practice and policy. Prospectively register evidence synthesis projects.
- Incorporate integrity assessment at every step of evidence synthesis (Box 9.5).
- Revisit the evidence syntheses if integrity concerns in the included trials are identified after publication of the reviews undertaken. The nature of the integrity concerns will determine the nature of the update required. The update may take the form of a retraction with a resubmission of an updated manu-

Corrigendum: A correction notice concerning a paper's version of record when the error(s) in the research work do not impact the main findings.

script (Box 9.4), a corrigendum, or letter to the editor with an update of the statistical synthesis (Box 2.4).

Writing tips for review authors

- **Title page:** Follow reporting guidelines and the journal's instructions.
- **Abstract:** Include a brief description of trial integrity assessments. Give prospective review registration details.
- **Introduction:** Describe the review priority. Justify the review in light of the existing evidence syntheses.
- **Methods:** Provide prospective review registration details. Thoroughly describe the integrity assessments at each step of the review (Box 9.5). If any planned review aspects were modified due to integrity concerns, describe this in methods.
- **Results, tables, and figures:** Ensure that tables, figures, and statistical results give complete and clear descriptions of the integrity assessments.
- **Discussion:** Ensure a full discussion of the clinical usefulness of the findings in the light of integrity assessments. Draw inferences moderated by the impact of the integrity assessments undertaken. When recommending further research, give specific advice concerning the design and conduct of future trials.
- **Funding disclosures:** Give a full account of direct funding to the work.
- **Conflicts of interest declarations:** Provide a full account of both financial and personal interests.
- **Appendices:** Provide the list of studies excluded due to integrity concerns. Share data, analysis code, and output.

Roles of institutions, funders, and journals

- Institutions, funders, journals, and other stakeholders in the research ecosystem have the responsibility to learn from integrity concerns captured in evidence syntheses and correct the scientific record accordingly, without placing theburden on reviewers to become whistleblowers.
- Funders should prioritize methodological developments required to underpin the incorporation of integrity assessments in evidence syntheses, such as the creation of unified platforms for retractions, corrigenda,expressions of concerns, validation of instruments and checklists, development of automation to support evidence synthesis, and more.

Conflicts of interest: Potential or perceived compromise in the objectivity or judgment of anyone involved in research and publication due to financial or personal (non-financial) interests. Failure of declaration is considered research misconduct.

Whistleblower: An individual, also known as the complainant, who reports a possible current or past breach of research integrity for misconduct investigation.

10 Investigating research misconduct allegations

Research integrity: Undertaking trials in accordance with ethical and professional principles and standards. Integrity failures may result from honest errors.

Whistleblower: An individual, also known as the complainant, who reports a possible current or past breach of research integrity for investigation.

Misconduct: Unethical or unprofessional behavior in research that is intentional, reckless, or negligent. Honest error is not misconduct.

Questionable research practices: Irresponsible research practices that are regarded as unethical or unprofessional but fall short of being considered misconduct.

Journal: An establishment composed of editors and other publishing staff who organize peer review of trial manuscripts and their publication.

Honesty is the best practice throughout the research lifecycle of a trial. Not all trials are created with equal rigor, and flawed trials can misguide evidence-based healthcare. Thus, institutions, funders, and journals should have publicly available research misconduct investigation policies. Anyone involved in research, including both trialists and participants, can raise complaints at any time during the trial lifecycle. Whistleblowing has a recognized role, protected by law. Upon receipt of a formal complaint, which may be made anonymously, a preliminary assessment of its merits is conducted. At this stage, the complaint may be dismissed, or it may proceed to a formal investigation, where the respondent trialist will be expected to provide a statement of defense. The investigation committee may appoint external independent experts to provide evidence. If the allegations are not upheld, and if it is further concluded that they are malicious, action may be taken against the whistleblower. Mistaken complaints made in good faith should be met with the necessary protections against retaliation. Honest errors leading to integrity flaws may result in remedial training for the respondent trialists. Findings of questionable research practices and misconduct could result in a range of sanctions, including but not limited to retractions and dismissal from employment.

Concerns about integrity flaws

Not all trials are designed, conducted, analyzed, and reported with equal rigor. During the course of the trial, a whistleblower might file a complain with the institution where the trial is taking place, or a research governance office audit or inspection may discover a concern (Box 10.1). Even participants may raise complaints, such as issues related to their informed consent (Chapter 4). Upon submission of the manuscript to a journal, editors and peer reviewers assessing trial manuscripts may have questions pertaining to trial integrity. They may seek explanations concerning compliance with ethical and professional principles and standards. Authors must address these concerns and revise the manuscript to the journal's satisfaction before it is accepted for publication. In journals that practice open peer review, the reviewers' reports and the authors' responses will be published alongside the revised accepted version of the manuscript (Chapter 7). If the journal becomes concerned about trial integrity during its assessment, it may raise the issue with the institution employing the authors. The journal may do this regardless of whether

DOI: 10.1201/9781003461401-10

the manuscript is accepted for publication. Preprints released alongside submitted manuscripts may also invite questions from readers other than the peer reviewers invited by journals (also called pre-review). Readers may direct their queries to the journals assessing the manuscripts, post them as comments on the preprint platforms, or they may contact the authors' institutions. Authors have the opportunity to address all the points raised ahead of publication.

Then comes post-publication peer review. Readers appraising published trials may have questions, and they have various avenues available for seeking clarification. They can raise concerns through the journal's correspondence or letters section. Authors are responsible for responding to these queries, and the journals publish the responses along with readers' letters. These published interactions may allow for a better interpretation of the published findings. The correspondence between readers and authors is cited along with the record of the original trial in electronic bibliographic databases. Together, these citations constitute the trial's published research record.

Readers may also directly engage the trial authors outside the publishing journal's standard mechanism for moderated interaction. Data sleuthing, where volunteer researchers or journalists report possible flaws in published studies via blogging and social media, is on the rise. They may raise questions via academic online platforms such as PubPeer (pubpeer.com). Sleuthing involves the use of validated tools (e.g., digital image forensics, plagiarism checks) as well as so far unvalidated methods to signpost the possibility of research integrity flaws. Systematic reviewers may also approach trialists for clarification as they may observe issues that cannot be resolved based on the published research record (Chapter 9). If authors' responses are unsatisfactory to the readers or those undertaking evidence syntheses, they can sometimes turn to formal complaints about irresponsible research conduct. These complaints may be made to the journal editor, who may forward them to the institutions where the trial in question took place, i.e., the authors' employers. Trialists may then have to face investigations to defend themselves against research misconduct allegations.

There is much confusion about definitions and procedures amongst all parties involved in research misconduct allegations, including those raising concerns, those assessing the concerns, those responding to allegations, and those investigating the allegations and responses to make final judgments. Institutions, as employers of trialists, have a role covering the entire lifecycle of the trial, up to its publication. This role focuses on research ethics and governance necessary for compliance with standards such as Good Research Practice in human clinical trials (GCP). Institutions typically have their own research integrity policies and procedures, which may operate under the umbrella of national research in-

Formal peer review: The evaluation of scientific manuscripts by others working in the same field, invited by journal editors, prior to acceptance for publication as definitive articles representing the version of record.

Committee on Publication Ethics (COPE): Issues guidance to journals on handling research misconduct allegations (publicationethics .org).

Data sleuthing: Post-publication investigation of possible research misconduct and questionable research practices by volunteer researchers.

Institution: A clinical academic organization, such as a university or a hospital, where trials take place.

Research governance: The system set up by institutions to oversee that the conduct of trials under their auspices are in compliance with regulations.

Box 10.1: How concerns about research integrity might arise

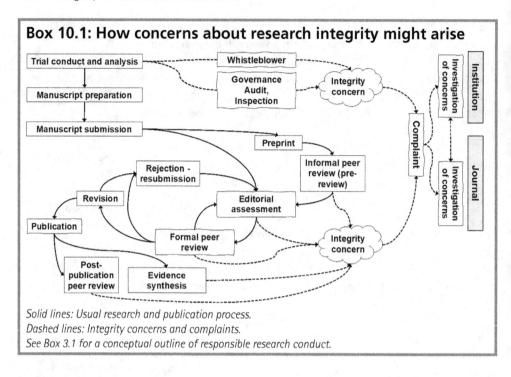

Solid lines: Usual research and publication process.
Dashed lines: Integrity concerns and complaints.
See Box 3.1 for a conceptual outline of responsible research conduct.

tegrity laws in some countries. Journals tend to become involved after a trial is completed, as they focus on the communication of information. Although they have the responsibility for ensuring that manipulation of peer review does occur, journals may not be best suited to address concerns raised about the trial's conduct itself. Journals and institutions should always cooperate in the handling of complaints about research integrity, but this does not always happen. Box 10.2 provides a brief outline of the classification of irresponsible research conduct, breaking integrity flaws down into research misconduct and questionable research practices. The term "research misconduct investigation" is used throughout this chapter to cover all allegations of irresponsible research conduct, including both misconduct and questionable practices.

Good Clinical Practice (GCP): A set of internationally recognized ethical and scientific quality standards for the design, conduct, recording, and analysis of randomized clinical trials.

Filing and assessing a complaint

Whistleblowing, i.e., drawing attention to wrongdoing to prevent societal harm, is protected by law. A whistleblower is an individual, also known as the complainant, who reports a possible current or past breach of research integrity. The term typically refers to issues arising in the workplace where both the complainant and the trialists are employed. Whistleblowers are usually outside observers, not directly involved in the trial. However, anyone directly involved in the research, including trialists

Trial: Throughout this book, the term "trial" refers to randomized clinical trials involving random allocation of eligible, consenting human participants to intervention groups and their follow-up to examine differences in group outcomes.

Box 10.2: Classification of irresponsible research conduct

Research misconduct
- Fabrication, Falsification, and Plagiarism (FFP).
- Ethical issues, such as failing to obtain human research ethics committee approval, failing to obtain informed consent, misinforming participants to obtain their consent, etc. (Chapter 4).
- Mismanagement of conflicts of interest.
- Breach of confidentiality.
- Unethical authorship, such as ghost authorship (not naming someone who meets authorship criteria), guest authorship (naming someone who does not meet authorship criteria), etc. (Chapter 8).
- Unethical publication practices, such as buying authorship through a paper mill, predatory publishing, etc. (Chapter 7).
- Publication process manipulation, such as organizing fake peer reviews, sharing peer-reviewed information with others, coercive citation practices, etc. (Chapter 7).
- Misconduct related to research misconduct investigation procedures.
- Misappropriating research funds and theft.
- Other deception or deviation.

Questionable research practices
- Spin in the description of research findings, including displaying misleading figures of data, such as truncating the axes to give a particular impression.
- Selective reporting of outcomes and manipulation of data analysis, such as p-hacking (Chapter 5).
- Self-plagiarism.
- Inadequate citation practices, such as unnecessary self-citation, inappropriate citations of others' works, and more.
- Authorship abuse, such as highly prolific authorship (without meeting authorship criteria), invented authorship (naming someone without their permission), and more (Chapter 8).
- Other irresponsible research practices.

Definitions and classifications vary across jurisdictions. Note that honest error is not misconduct.
See Box 3.1 for the relation between various terms and practices related to responsible research conduct.
See Box 10.4 for some basic points about conducting investigations into allegations of research misconduct.
Sources: DOI's: 10.1080/08989621.2014.958218; 10.1177/1747016119898400.

and participants, can also raise complaints at any time during the trial lifecycle. Research misconduct and questionable research practices can affect study participants and may have downstream consequences for healthcare practice and policy. They can also damage the work environment or research culture in institutions where trials take place (Chapter 3). Institutions should have a publicly available whistleblowing policy.

The whistleblower provides written notification of a suspected case of research misconduct or questionable research practice to the organization with an investigative role, such as an institution, journal, funder, professional regulatory body, etc. This notification is sometimes also known as a formal complaint. Depending on the policies, complaints can be lodged anonymously. Even if not lodged anonymously, the whistleblower has the right to anonymity and confidentiality during the proceedings. Whistleblowers are meant to be protected against retaliation, which is particularly important as junior staff tend to be vulnerable against powerful senior researchers. Without protection, they may not come forward. Confidentiality serves to help achieve this objective. If identified, whistleblowers may face backlash, such as workplace stigma, suffer in career progression, or may even lose their employment or research funding. Data sleuthing typically lacks protections in the same way as whistleblowing at the workplace has. Sleuths typically raise complaints publicly and may face legal threats. To defend themselves, they may be able to access legal services pro bono or through legal aid if their claims are assessed to be made in good faith. Otherwise, they may have to finance their defense themselves or through crowdfunding.

Whistleblowers tend to believe strongly in the merit of their complaint. They may demand that the investigation should be opened to them, especially if they feel that their complaint is not being taken seriously or if they do not have confidence in the competence of investigators. This is not the norm. Other than reporting their complaint, whistleblowers should not take any further part in investigations. Disgruntled whistleblowers, especially in cases where the investigation outcome favors respondent trialists, may resort to repeating their complaints in other forums. This may amount to defamation, especially when there is no case to answer on the assessment on the merits of the complaint or the conclusion of a research misconduct investigation. They may first complain to journals, then to institutions. They may also go public, risking a breach of confidentiality in misconduct investigations. Courts have been known to award substantial damages for defamation against complainants who violate confidentiality. See the case study in Box 10.3. However annoying it may be to become the subject of a complaint or repeated complaints, honest trialists should remain calm and work within the limits of their institutional research integrity policies.

Complaints must be made in good faith, and supported by evidence of wrongdoing or strong suspicion. The first task of an investigation officer or committee is to make a preliminary assessment if this is the case. For this, they should examine the evidence on which the research misconduct allegation is based. They may ask the whistleblower to provide more information, including any analysis codes and outputs. A bad-faith

Confidentiality: Keeping disclosed information private. In research misconduct investigations, disclosure is made only on a need-to-know basis. A breach of confidentiality is a form of research misconduct.

Power: The ability to influence others. The role asymmetry in a relationship permits the powerful to influence the vulnerable. The responsibility to prevent influence from turning into abuse lies with the powerful party.

Trialist: An investigator who contributes to a trial and is credited in the authorship or the acknowledgment section of the published article.

Respondent: The trialist whose research conduct is the subject of a complaint or is being investigated.

Policy: A guideline or set of rules.

Procedure: Step-by-step instructions for implementing a policy.

Box 10.3: Case study – $160 thousand compensation for a doctoral student in a defamation claim against the professor

- A doctoral research student sued her professor for defamation in a court case.
- The professor had made research misconduct allegations against the student in a formal complaint to the university.
- The university's research integrity office, in its initial assessment of the merits of the complaint, concluded that there was not sufficient evidence to initiate a research misconduct investigation.
- The professor was instructed to keep his concerns about research misconduct confidential.
- However, the professor continued to express his concerns about the student's research misconduct to colleagues and family members who had no formal role in handling the complaint he had made.
- The jury concluded that the student's reputation was damaged by the professor's confidentiality breach.
- The student was awarded $160,000 in compensation.

Source: United States District Court, District of Utah Case number 2:15-CV-767-TS.
URL: storage.courtlistener.com/recap/gov.uscourts.utd.98282/gov.uscourts.utd.98282.237.0.pdf.

complaint may be filed for the purpose of harming the trialist, and it may be insignificant in its substance. There are many published "red flags" for distinguishing researcher harassment from genuine concerns. There cannot be an investigation of a complaint that merely reflects a difference of scientific opinion. If the allegation made is found to be malicious, disciplinary proceedings may be initiated against the whistleblower in some circumstances. If the whistleblower has waited too long since publication (a 5 or 10-year time limit may apply), they should provide justification for a late complaint; otherwise, it is typically thrown out. To make their assessment, the investigation committee may seek to have sight of the whistleblower's own record. The complaint history may reveal that it is a repeat complaint. The whistleblower may be asked to declare conflicts of interests, in the same way as authors do when submitting papers. If the complaint is found to be meritorious, an investigation will commence.

Unfortunately, it is a common experience that many of those who initially assess the allegations lack the competence to determine whether the complaint is meritorious or whether there is no case to answer. They may also be under pressure, given that the consequences of a finding of misconduct may lead to the retraction of papers, which in turn may affect their organization's reputation. The current culture of science means that those assessing complaints are more likely to err on the side of caution. They may initiate investigations, regardless of the strength of the evidence underpinning the concerns raised. This means that even in

Conflicts of interest: Potential or perceived compromise in the objectivity or judgment of anyone involved in research misconduct investigation due to financial or personal (non-financial) interests. Failure of declaration is considered research misconduct.

Retraction: The removal of a published paper from the research record, for example, due to the discovery of a flaw in its integrity.

cases of flimsy allegations, honest trialists are likely to find themselves in the dock defending themselves.

Formal research misconduct investigation

The investigating organization may be an institution, journal, funder, or another organization. When allegations are assessed to have merit on initial screening, a formal misconduct investigation is triggered in accordance with the organization's research integrity policies and procedures. Depending on the nature of the complaint, it may be passed between organizations, such as a journal may pass it to the institution for investigation. In some circumstances, such as when journals do not trust institutions, as could happen when the two parties are in different geographical jurisdictions. They may insist on reaching their own conclusions, even if the institutions say that there is no case to answer.

Only trialists who are or were under contract with an organization to undertake and publish research can be subjected to investigations. There does not need to be a written employment contract, as an implied contract can be deemed to exist due to the trialist's participation in an approved trial. Even if the trialist has left the organization before the allegations are made, the organization may still be obliged to investigate. This is because institutions, journals, funders, and other organizations involved in trials must take responsibility for any research performed and published under their auspices. They may even waive time limitations under some circumstances. It is important to recognize that institutions, journals, and funders have potential conflicts of interest when investigating their own employees, authors, and funded investigators. This could be in favor of or against the respondent trialist. To ensure objectivity, it would be better that an independent or external organization, such as a national research integrity body or another institution, journal, or funder not involved in the research, to investigate allegations of irresponsible research conduct. However, this is not the current practice. It has been argued that the organizations directly involved in the research and its publication should restrict themselves to investigating allegations that fall in the category of questionable research practices, while research misconduct investigations should be handled externally.

Procedures in investigations vary between organizations, and Box 10.4 provides some generic basic points that apply in brief. The organization must follow its research integrity policies and procedures when conducting an investigation. Their decisions may be appealed in national research integrity bodies, where such structure exist, or in courts of law. Upon determining that the allegation is meritorious, an investigation committee

Box 10.4: Some basic points about research misconduct investigations

General

- Institutions, journals, and funders should have a publicly available research misconduct investigation policy.
- Honest error is not misconduct.
- All parties involved in an investigation, including both whistleblowers and respondent trialists, have a duty to maintain confidentiality.
- The professional standards for judgment are those prevailing at the time of the alleged research misconduct.
- Very old complaints, e.g., 5 or 10 years after publication, are not investigated.
- Investigations must be fair, managing conflicts of interest and respecting equality and diversity regulations. Independent or external organizations may be better placed to undertake investigations more objectively.
- The investigation timeline should follow strict deadlines for its various stages, in accordance with the policy and procedures for research misconduct investigation.
- Investigation procedures for financial fraud or other researcher misconduct may be handled through a disciplinary policy different from the research integrity policy.

Whistleblower

- To trigger an investigation, complaints must be assessed to have been made in good faith with reasonable belief or evidence of wrongdoing.
- Whistleblowers have the right to anonymity.
- Whistleblowers do not take an active part in investigations other than reporting their complaint.
- Whistleblowers have the right to protection against retaliation.

Respondent trialists

- Respondents have the right to the presumption of innocence.
- Respondents have a right to know the exact allegations made.
- Respondents have the right to be informed about the process and the stage of the procedure at any time during the investigation.
- Respondent trialists have the right to protection against double jeopardy, i.e., being subjected to investigation twice for the same misconduct allegation, particularly when a previous investigation has found no case to answer.
- Respondents have the right to review the evidence and to interview witnesses, with or without the input of a legal counsel.

Findings and sanctions

- The judgments in investigations are made based on the balance of probability, i.e., over 50% likelihood, not based on "beyond reasonable doubt".

- A distinction should be made between the integrity flaw found and whether or not this resulted from misconduct.
- In case of honest errors, remedial training should be considered as part of any sanctions.
- The decisions of investigations can be challenged in national integrity forums where they exist or in courts of law.

Procedures vary across jurisdictions; the term "research misconduct investigation" covers all allegations of irresponsible research conduct, including both misconduct and questionable practices outlined in Box 10.2.
See Box 3.1 for an outline of the relation between various terms and practices related to responsible research conduct and research misconduct investigations.

is typically appointed. At this point, the journal that published the trial in question may issue an expression of concern. Theoretically, this is not a statement of scientific misconduct (an exoneration statement will have to be issued if there was no misconduct found upon completion of the investigation). However, this has reputational implications. Trialists may seek the assistance from the courts to prevent the publication of a notice of expression of concern. Courts are known to intervene to protect the accused scientist's reputation at this stage. Respondent trialists have the right to the presumption of innocence.

The investigation committee will consist of a chair and several individual members. They may or may not have taken part in the initial assessment of the complaint. Ideally, committee members should have research competence and no link to the whistleblower or the respondent. If several organizations are involved, each may nominate their own members. Management of committee conflicts of interest can be challenging, but openness in this regard is key to a fair investigation. The investigation must be free of outside interference from parties with vested interests in a particular outcome, and it must be perceived as such The committee composition and choice of experts must also respect equality and diversity regulations. The possibility of discrimination, such as violation of the right to protection against bias and harm arising on account of differences in gender, race, religion, disability, sexual orientation, and more, is real in organizations that are not conscious of their social responsibilities. The academic landscape is known to be polluted by bias in this respect at all levels including appointments, promotions, research funding, peer review, and disciplinary procedures are likely to be no exception.

Often, the complainant makes multiple allegations at once, and not all the individual allegations may be meritorious. The respondent has the right to be informed of the allegations that will be pursued in the

Expression of concern: A note published by a journal to inform readers of a potential concern about the integrity of a paper.

Equality: People should not be disadvantaged because of differences in gender, race, religion, disability, sexual orientation, or other protected characteristics.

Discrimination: The result of applying policies and practices to some individuals but not to others based on their protected characteristics.

investigation. Making the determination as to which allegations to pursue and which to discard is not an easy task. Frequently, the investigation committee will pass on the complaint document submitted by the whistleblower in its entirety to the respondent (care should be taken to help maintain anonymity, such as redacting the whistleblower's identity). A lack of specification in the allegations being pursued could be a sign of committee incompetence or inexperience. Respondent trialists have the right to transparency and to be informed of the specific allegations. They may need to ask the investigation committee to clarify exactly what will be investigated. The committee should apply the organization's policies and procedures strictly, otherwise they risk losing the case on appeal for failure to follow the procedures.

The investigation committee will seek a response to the complaint from respondent trialists. This is the statement of defense. The trialist may be interviewed. The committee may also seek expert evidence from someone independent and competent in the field. It may conduct its own data reanalysis if its members have the competence to do so. In many countries, institutions are required by law to retain study data for a period of time after the completion of research, so they may have the trial dataset available for reanalysis. There may be hearings where cross-examination of the witnesses takes place regarding their evidence. The hearings may be audio recorded or transcribed.

The committee will evaluate all material collated in the investigation to come up with its findings regarding the misconduct allegation. In theory, the finding should be evidence-based and judged using the preponderance of evidence or the balance of probabilities rule, i.e., more than 50% probability (note how vastly different it is from the 95% probability threshold, i.e., $p < 0.05$, used in scientific hypothesis testing). This is not an easy decision, as the judgment involves determining not only that misconduct took place, but also that it was intentional, committed knowingly, or recklessly (Box 3.1). Investigation findings should make a distinction between establishing whether an integrity breach took place, and whether this occurred as a result of deliberate misconduct. Honest error is not misconduct. Most investigation committee members have no legal training. They may not even be trialists or scientists in the same field or discipline, so they may lack relevant experience. Even in straightforward cases, coming up with findings will involve considerable exercise of judgment to determine which way the case goes on the preponderance of evidence.

The final report of the investigation, which usually contains the case in its entirety, including the allegations, the defense, the evidence, the expert reports, the justification for the decision, the decision, and the recommendations, is meant to be treated as confidential in perpetu-

Balance of probabilities: Proving that something is more likely than not to have happened, i.e., over 50% probability.

ity. Where investigation reports have been made public, such as in legal challenges to the institutional investigation outcome, these have been noted to be quite sizeable documents, sometimes running into hundreds of pages. In theory, regardless of the outcome of the investigation, none of the parties involved should make further comment after the case is closed. Given human nature, this is easier said than done. In any case, as expressions of concern, exoneration notices, and retractions may be involved, the word gets out. News media may take an interest in such cases and they tend to have no difficulty in finding informants.

Respondent trialists

Given the bar for decision-making is only at the level of balance of probabilities, not at the "beyond reasonable doubt" standard of proof, the stakes are high. For an honest trialist, the risk of being falsely accused in research misconduct investigations exists. It is important to emphasize that the scientific standard of proof ($p < 0.05$ or 95% probability threshold) is not applied in misconduct investigations. Trialists should thus take the investigations very seriously. The scenario is set for the need to seek legal counsel. This is normally permitted, and should not be taken as a sign that the respondent has something to hide. Trialists may also instruct their own expert witnesses. The involvement of a counsel may increase the likelihood that the investigation will be conducted by the policies and procedure, or at least, if this is not the case, the counsel will be able to address this matter.

The respondent trialist should prepare the statement of defense thoroughly, just as they would prepare a scientific paper or a research grant application with time and effort. They must strictly meet all deadlines. If this is not possible, they need to formally seek deadline extensions There is a possibility that during the investigation the trialist may be excluded from the workplace (also known as suspension). In this case, they will be unable to examine the records kept at the office. They must seek official permission to obtain whatever information they need from the workplace to prepare their defense thoroughly. Their counsel may have to request access formally. The trialists should take the opportunity to cross-examine the witnesses, including expert witnesses appointed by the committee. They must carefully take their own notes in any interviews and hearings. Sometimes, they may be permitted to have the support of a colleague, who may be able to take notes on their behalf.

In addition to their statement of defense, trialists may be able to make further submissions as the proceedings go forward. They must review the transcripts of all interviews and hearings to ensure they have been correctly recorded. The administrative staff assisting investigators may not be up to the mark as they might lack training in the task. Trialists may even make their own audio recordings with permission. The errors in transcripts of the interviews and hearings should be pointed out, as the investigation committee would likely rely on these, instead of their own memory or notes, when making decisions. If necessary, the trialists also have the rights under freedom of information laws to make requests to obtain information about themselves that may not have been supplied in the investigation. Any organization that may hold any recorded data, including e-mails, letters, handwritten notes, audio recordings, or videos of meetings, concerning the trialist, is obligated to hand it over within specified time limits. Trialists should review all the evidence in front of the committee and submit their own analysis backed by their own notes. The committee has the obligation to evaluate all alternative interpretations of the evidence before reaching a final decision.

> **Freedom of information:** The right of individuals to access information that pertains to them.

To undertake the defense in a legally robust manner will help in case the trialists have to appeal the decision of the investigation. This may have to be in a national research integrity forum, or a court of law.

Sanctions

Hopefully, there will be no surprises for innocent trialists. With some luck, there will be no case for them to answer on the preliminary assessment of the complaints made. If the matter progresses, they should be cleared by competent, unbiased investigations. The investigation report, i.e., its parts that others need to know, should be shared between stakeholder organizations, e.g., an institutional investigation should share its findings with relevant journals and funders. In the case where any expression of concern notices have been initially published, these would need to be followed up by the publication of exoneration statements. While journals are quick to post concern notices, they may not be so active in publishing exoneration statements. Trialists may have to actively insist on getting the investigation outcomes published to clear their names. In case honest errors are found, journals have the option to publish a corrigendum. They also have the option to retract and republish. There are many examples of this, such as a trial where a randomization error is found, can be reanalyzed and published as an observational cohort study. Honest error may also be indicate a need for training. The reason for a flaw in research integrity could very well be a trialist's lack of research ability, and looking at the issue this way may help identify learning needs. Engagement in a relevant educational program leading to error avoidance will protect the integrity of future research projects. Another important consideration for research integrity investigators is determining the contribution of the workplace culture in their assessments. Feedback should be provided to

> **Corrigendum:** A correction notice concerning a paper's version of record when the error(s) in the research work do not impact on the main findings.

organizational directors. Lessons learned through investigations should lead to concrete organizational actions that help drive continuous improvements in the research culture.

If a finding of misconduct is made in an investigation, sanctions will follow accordingly. Different organizations may impose various sanctions. The trial publication may be retracted by the journal, or a corrigendum may be published. If the retracted research is associated with the award of a qualification or degree, such as a PhD, it may be withdrawn subject to further investigation by the degree-awarding university. There may be a research or publication ban placed for a period of time. The research funding may be withdrawn or a funding ban placed. There may be loss of employment or demotion. If employment is maintained, there may be retraining requirements that would have to be met through a tailored professional development plan and demonstrable evidence of researcher behavior correction to bring it in line with research integrity principles. If the professional regulatory body of the trialist is informed, e.g., in the case of a researcher who is a licened healthcare practitioner, there may be further fitness-to-practice proceedings. This will take its course and there may be a period of suspension, corrective training with reinstatement of licence, or removal from the practitioner register. The outcomes of professional regulatory body investigations can be challenged in the law courts. Have a look at the case study in Box 10.5.

The outcomes of research misconduct investigations can be challenged in national integrity forums where they exist or in courts of law. National research integrity policies should be consolidated within an international framework as randomized clinical trials and the use of their findings in healthcare are truly a global affair.

Professional regulatory body: By law, healthcare professionals must be registered with a professional regulatory body to ensure they are fit and licensed to practice. It may undertake a fitness-to-practice investigation upon being alerted about a research integrity concern. (Note: The term "regulator" used in this book is different as it is a formal body set up for official approvals of medicines and devices, such as the European Medicines Agency).

Correcting the research record for societal benefit

The research record consists of accepted manuscripts in their definitive form called the version of record. The process of record correction can begin as soon as a complaint about a published trial is considered meritorious. At this stage, an expression of concern may be issued by the journal, notifying of a research misconduct allegation, unless authors are able to prevent this from happening by convincing the journal to wait or by taking the judicial route. This notice is just a stopgap until the misconduct investigation comes up with some findings. While the expression of concern is active, it is unlikely that the trial in question will be used; for example, evidence syntheses may discard them (Chapter 9). If there is no case to answer, a formal letter including an apology is issued to the trialists by the investigating journal or institution. If an expression

Version of record: The final published version of the manuscript in its definitive form with copyediting and typesetting completed, metadata applied, and a DOI (digital object identifier) allocated.

of concern was initially published, the next record correction stage is the publication of an exoneration statement. If this cycle takes too long, genuine trial findings may remain out of circulation, failing to realize the societal benefit expected through the healthcare research pursuit. This will reverse the efforts of all those working to promote the evidence-based medicine paradigm.

In cases of minor errors, a correction notice in the form of a corrigendum may be published. This is the case when the interpretation of the trial may be slightly affected, but the research integrity and main trial findings are intact. Trialists may request this at any time without the need to wait for a formal complaint, or the findings of an investigation. The error may not be readily classified as minor or major. Dealing with this situation via an extensive correction leaves the research record in a grey area. Retraction, the dreaded tool for correcting the research record, is used to correct a major error that invalidates the main trial findings due to an honest error, or research misconduct and questionable research practices (Box 10.2). The retraction may be author-requested, or it may be the result of the findings of a research misconduct investigation by the institution, journal, or another stakeholder organization. Retractions carry a stigma, even though they are intended to correct the research record. Part of their stigmatic nature comes from the fact that journals usually do not report clear-cut reasons for the retraction. The online version of the retracted citation contains the retraction notice and its version of record is watermarked with the word "retracted". Although the online version of the paper may be removed, the citation and the version of record remain available in perpetuity. For those browsing, it may raise suspicion affecting the reputation of trialists. See a case study of a retraction of an interpretation followed by a full article retraction in Box 10.5. There have been calls for changes in research record correction towards more responsible post-publication practices.

In cases of major errors where the data remain genuine, retraction should be associated with republication. Obviously, in cases of fraudulent misconduct such as falsification or fabrication, no republication is justified. If such fatal flaws are excluded, retraction with republication should become the norm. For example, when the data are genuine but there is some other design or analysis flaw, such as faulty randomization or statistics, republication is justified. The journal should encourage the republication of the study with major corrections implemented, such as considering a study with faulty randomization as an observational cohort study and republishing it as such. In this situation, the corrected paper will need substantial changes, such as instead of CONSORT, it will need to follow the STROBE reporting checklist, a multivariable analysis will be required to control for confounding, and more. When republish-

Evidence-based medicine: The conscientious, explicit, and judicious use of current best research evidence in making healthcare decisions.

EQUATOR: A network for improving health research reporting (equator-network.org).

CONSORT: Consolidated Standards of Reporting Trials.

STROBE: STrengthening the Reporting of OBservational studies in Epidemiology.

ing, the paper will need to pass editorial and peer review assessment on resubmission, and the associated retraction notice should be transparent. As evidence-based medicine ranks cohort studies next in the evidence hierarchy after randomized clinical trials, there is no reason why such evidence should be lost forever through retraction without republication. This approach will also help encourage trialists to come forward spontaneously or when prompted in cases of honest errors, especially if institutions and funders ensure that honest trialists' careers are not affected. Who knows, one day, retraction with republication may even become the hallmark of a credible trialist. The research record correction is a murky landscape that needs much redesigning work to continue promoting research integrity.

Box 10.5: Case study – Retraction of an article triggered by a fitness-to-practice investigation

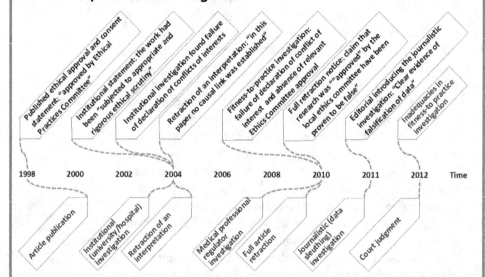

- A 1998 article became central to a UK child vaccination scandal.
- In 2004, an institutional (university/hospital) investigation of misconduct allegations identified a failure to declare conflicts of interest, and stated that the work published had been "subjected to appropriate and rigorous ethical scrutiny".
- On the same date as the publication of the institutional reply in 2004, a retraction of an interpretation by an author subgroup stated that "in this paper, no causal link was established" between the vaccine exposure and the outcome.
- A subsequent fitness-to-practice investigation undertaken by the medical professional regulator of some co-authors concluded in 2010. It agreed with the institutional investigation on the failure to declare a conflict of interest but disagreed concerning ethics committee approval.

- The journal retracted the article fully in 2010 as the institutional claims that the research published was "'approved' by the local ethics committee have been proven to be false" in the fitness-to-practice investigation.
- A 2011 editorial in another journal claimed that there was "evidence of falsification of data" based on sleuthing by a journalist who had compared the documents made public by the fitness-to-practice investigation with the findings reported in the 1998 article. Coincidentally, a corrigendum to the editorial admitted its own failure to declare financial conflicts of interest due to receiving "advertising and sponsorship revenue from vaccine manufacturers".
- Questions remain about how the institution and the professional regulator came to decide differently on the status of the ethics committee approval. Moreover, the deliberations of the professional regulator were found to be inadequate in a 2012 court judgment.
- The 1998 paper remains retracted without any changes to the 2010 retraction notice.

There are many aspects to this complex case study. The above is a brief and simplified outline highlighting the issues related to ethical approval, failure of declaration of conflicts of interest, the multiplicity of research misconduct investigations, and the retraction of an interpretation followed by full retraction. Source: DOI's: 10.1016/S0140-6736(10)60175-4; 10.1016/S0140-6736(04)15699-7; 10.1016/S0140-6736(04)15715-2; 10.1136/bmj.c7452. URL's: bailii.org/ew/cases/EWHC/Admin/2012/503.html; pubpeer.com/publications/CF52AD098D3AC46 2697D50B97B3105.

Chapter 10: Investigating research misconduct allegations – Key points

Handling integrity concerns raised (advice to respondent trialists)

- Plan, execute, and report trials with the highest possible level of transparency as a preventive measure against complaints.
- Stay up-to-date with the research training requirements, such as GCP certification and consent training.
- Respond to all queries whether before or post-publication fully and honestly (an honest error is not misconduct). Respond to comments on social media platforms while respecting confidentiality and institutional research integrity policies and procedures.
- Take research misconduct investigations seriously, responding to concerns raised fully and honestly. Engage a counsel in the preparation of the statement of defense, if required.

Transparency in research: Open research practices, including prospective registration, adherence to trial design, *a priori* statistical analysis plan, data sharing, and timely and complete public reporting.

- Retain datasets securely in accordance with the law in case they may be required for future defense in research misconduct investigations.
- Fully undertake any remedial training required at the conclusion of a research misconduct investigation.
- If required, actively engage with journals in the publication of expressions of concern and exoneration notices, and in correcting the research record through retraction, republication, etc.

Roles of institutions, journals, and funders

- Institutions, journals, funders, and other stakeholder organizations, such as professional societies, should have a publicly available research misconduct investigation policy. All stakeholder organizations regardless of country jurisdictions should work towards achieving harmonization of research integrity policies and procedures (Chapter 3).
- Institutions should implement strong research governance to audit compliance with regulations, such as GCP. Prevention of misconduct is better than the need for investigation and subsequent research record correction.
- Institutions should establish the infrastructure required to retain datasets in accordance with the law. Data may be required for any re-examination in research misconduct investigations.
- Journals should appoint a research integrity editor and implement a research integrity training program for their staff. Prevention is better than cure: Journals should publish trials responsibly, investing in proper prepublication assessment to minimize retraction risk (Chapter 7).
- Institutions and journals should cooperate in misconduct investigations, including complaints about inadequate consent (Chapter 4) and unethical authorship (Chapter 8). Timeliness is a key factor. Institutions and journals should have mutual agreements for sharing confidential information on a need-to-know basis.
- Institutions and journals should protect whistleblowers and make whistleblowing policies publicly available.
- Ideally, independent or external organizations not involved in the trial conduct and its publication should undertake any investigations of alleged research misconduct.

Societies: Non-profit organizations that seek to further a particular healthcare profession and the interests of their patients.

Authorship abuse: Unethical authorship including naming authors not strictly based on contribution, such as guest authorship, ghost authorship, invented authorship, and more (Box 8.3).

- Research misconduct investigations, whether conducted by institutions, journals, or other bodies, should be fair and they should be seen to be fair. Only complaints made in good faith, based on evidence or strong suspicion, should be investigated. The procedures followed should observe key features such as presumption of innocence, maintenance of confidentiality, and protection of anonymity. Investigations should be free of conflicts of interest and mindful of equality, diversity, and inclusion issues. Investigation findings should make a distinction between establishing whether an integrity breach took place, and whether this occurred as a result of honest error or intentional, knowing, or reckless misconduct. Sanctions should focus on the correction of the research record and remedial training.

- Lessons learned from research misconduct investigations should be employed to make concrete changes in the workplace to continuously improve the research culture.

Research culture: The academic environment comprising of the norms, values, expectations, attitudes, and behaviors within research organizations. Academic freedom, collegiality, collaboration, equality and diversity, research integrity (ethics and professionalism), openness, and transparency are all features of the research culture.

Suggested reading

This book focuses on core information about randomized clinical trial integrity. It relies on the evidence gathered for undertaking the following works co-authored with colleagues who collectively have expertise across the entire lifecycle of trials. The reference lists of these articles provide a rich and comprehensive bibliography consolidating a diverse body of literature scattered across many disciplines.

- The quality and reporting of recommendation documents to enhance the integrity of clinical trials: a systematic review and critical appraisal. Semergen 2024, accepted paper awaiting DOI allocation at the time of book publication.
- Post-publication research integrity concerns in randomized clinical trials: A scoping review of the literature. Int J Gynaecol Obstet 2024;166:984–993. DOI: 10.1002/ijgo.15488.
- Research integrity in randomised clinical trials: a scoping umbrella review. Int J Gynaecol Obstet 2023;162:860–876. DOI: 10.1002/ijgo.14762.
- International multi-stakeholder consensus statement on clinical trial integrity. BJOG 2023;13:1096–1111. DOI: 10.1111/1471-0528.17451.
- Assessing the integrity of clinical trials included in evidence syntheses. Int J Environ Res Public Health 2023;20:6138. DOI: 10.3390/ijerph20126138.
- Assessing the usefulness of randomised trials in obstetrics and gynaecology. BJOG 2023;30:695–701. DOI: 10.1111/1471-0528.17411.
- Integrity of randomized clinical trials: Performance of integrity tests and checklists requires assessment. Int J Gynaecol Obstet 2023;163:733–743. DOI: 10.1002/ijgo.14837.
- Benefits of participation in clinical trials: an umbrella review. Int J Environ Res Public Health 2022;19:15368. DOI: 10.3390/ijerph192215368.
- Research integrity in clinical trials: innocent errors and spin versus scientific misconduct. Curr Opin Obstet Gynecol 2022;34:332–339. DOI: 10.1097/GCO.0000000000000807.

There is a need for harmonization of definitions for the various stakeholders responsible for randomized clinical trial integrity to speak the same language. So this book provides a detailed Glossary of terms. The sources of definitions consulted are listed below:

- Glossary. Systematic Reviews to Support Evidence-Based Medicine. How to Appraise, Conduct and Publish Reviews. 3rd Edition. London: Taylor & Francis Publishing, 2022:193–206. DOI: 10.1201/9781003220039.
- Glossary for Research and Academic Ethics and Integrity. Available at https://h2020integrity .eu/resources/glossary/.
- The Health Technology Assessment (HTA) glossary. Available at https://htaglossary.net.
- The European Medicines Agency (EMA) glossary. Available at https://www.ema.europa.eu/en/ about-us/glossaries/glossary-regulatory-terms.
- The National Institute for Health and Care Research (NIHR) glossary. Available at https://www .nihr.ac.uk/glossary.
- The ClinicalTrials.gov glossary. Available at https://www.clinicaltrials.gov/study-basics/glossary.

Glossary

This glossary uses information from the publications listed in the Suggested Reading section. The definitions provided here are those used in this book.

ACTIVE : A framework for citizen (and other stakeholder) involvement in evidence syntheses (Authors and Consumers Together Impacting on eVidencE, DOI: 10.1177/1355819619841647). *Also see* **GRIPP** and **Open Science**.

Adaptive trial : *See* **Platform trial**.

Adverse event : It is an undesirable and unintended harmful or unpleasant occurrence associated with an intervention. If there is a suggestion of a causal relationship, then the term used is adverse reaction. It may warrant prevention or specific treatment or alteration or withdrawal of the intervention. *Also see* **Outcome adjudication committee** and **Withdrawal**.

AGREE II : The second version of AGREE (Appraisal of Guidelines for REsearch and Evaluation), an instrument for evaluating the quality and reporting of clinical practice guidelines (agreetrust.org/agree-ii). *Also see* **RIGHT** and **Clinical practice guideline**.

AllTrials : A campaign for all past and present clinical trials to be registered and their methods and summary results reported (alltrials.net). *Also see* **RIAT**.

AMSTAR-2 : The second version of AMSTAR (A MeaSurement Tool to Assess systematic Reviews), an instrument for evaluating the quality of systematic reviews (amstar.ca). *Also see* **ROBIS**.

Applicability (external validity or **generalizability)** : The extent to which the effects of the trial intervention can be expected to apply in routine clinical practice, i.e., in those for whom the intervention is intended but who did not or could not participate in the trial. *Also see* **Validity (internal), Effectiveness** and **Efficacy**.

Applied research : Motivated by the desire to be useful in solving real-world problems, applied research aims to provide solutions. *Also see* **Basic research** and **Usefulness of research**.

Arm : A group of participants in a randomized clinical trial that receives a specific intervention according to the approved trial protocol. The trial arm may receive an active intervention, a control intervention, no intervention, a placebo, etc. A two-arm trial has two groups, one that receives the new intervention and another that receives a control intervention usually based on standard of care. A multi-arm trial has several intervention groups. *Also see* **Randomized clinical trial, Multi-arm multistage trial, Intervention** and **Randomization**.

Artificial intelligence (AI) : Automated solutions, using methods like machine learning, natural language processing, data mining, information retrieval and other computer science methods, to perform tasks that usually require human intelligence (language understanding, reasoning, learning, etc.). Traditional AI processes data to give results or predictions, e.g., plagiarism checks are automated. Unlike generative AI, traditional AI does not produce new content. *Also see* **Generative artificial intelligence (AI)**.

Attrition bias (exclusion bias) : Systematic differences between trial groups caused by exclusion or dropout of participants (e.g., because of side-effects of intervention) from the trial. Intention-to-treat analysis in combination with appropriate sensitivity analyses including all participants can protect against this bias. *Also see* **Intention-to-treat (ITT) analysis** and **Withdrawals.**

Audit : A planned formal evaluation of trial conduct, i.e., activities, such as informed consent, and documents, such as data collection and recording, to independently determine if the trial is being undertaken according to its approved protocol, and if it meets professional standards such as Good Clinical Practice in human clinical trials (GCP). *Also see* **Inspection**, **Forensic statistical analysis, GCP, Ethics** and **Research governance.**

Authorship : Giving credit to those who design, conduct, analyze and report a trial, i.e., naming those who have made substantial contributions to the work leading to the completion of the trial. Authors are accountable for the trial in its published form. *Also see* **Unethical authorship, ICMJE** and **CRediT.**

Authorship abuse : *See* **Unethical authorship, Guest authorship, Collaboration authorship, Convenience authorship, Ghost authorship, Orphan authorship,** and **Invented authorship.**

Autonomy : The fundamental research ethics principle that potential participants should make their own, independent, informed and entirely voluntary decision to sign up for a trial. *Also see* **Ethics, Moral values,** and **Human research ethics committee.**

Auto-plagiarism : *See* **Plagiarism.**

Balance of probabilities : Proving that something is more likely than not to have happened, i.e., over 50% probability. This is the standard of proof used in cases of research misconduct investigations. This is in sharp contrast to the 'beyond reasonable doubt' yardstick applied in criminal cases in courts. Also note how vastly different the balance of probabilities rule is from the 95% probability threshold, $p < 0.05$, used in scientific hypothesis testing.

Baseline risk : *See* **Prognosis.**

Basic research : Motivated by curiosity, basic research aims to generate new knowledge. *Also see* **Applied research** and **Usefulness of research.**

Bench-to-bedside : *See* **Research translation.**

Beneficence : The fundamental research ethics principle that trials ought to be undertaken for societal benefit. Benefits may also arise for participants through the process of taking part in a trial and this ought to be balanced against the potential risks. *Also see* **Ethics, Moral values,** and **Human research ethics committee.**

Bias (systematic error) : A tendency for trial results to depart systematically, either lower or higher, from the 'true' results. Bias either exaggerates or underestimates the 'true' effect of an intervention. Bias may arise due to systematic differences in comparison groups (selection bias), differences in care or exposure to factors other than the intervention of interest (performance bias), differences in assessment of outcomes (measurement bias), withdrawals or exclusions of participants enrolled into the trial (attrition bias), etc. Trials with unbiased results are said to be internally valid. Bias is distinct from research integrity flaws that arise due to misconduct or questionable research practices. *Also see* **Validity (internal validity)** and **Random error**.

Binary data : Measurement where the data have one of two alternatives, e.g., the patient is either alive or dead, the adverse event is present or absent, etc. For binary data, the effect is often expressed in terms of relative risk. *Also see* **Continuous data**.

Blinding (masking) : Blinding keeps the trial participants and trialists (including clinical investigators and outcome assessors) ignorant about the group allocation. In single-blind trials only the participants are ignorant about their group allocation, whilst in double-blind studies both the participants and trialists are blind. Outcome assessors can often be blinded even when participants and trialists can't be. Blinding protects against performance bias and detection bias, and it may contribute to adequate allocation concealment during randomization. *Also see* **Randomization**.

Case report form : A paper-based or electronic document used for data collection from each consenting participant in a trial. Once collected, the data are entered into the trial database used for statistical analysis and reporting. The protection of participant privacy and confidentiality are key issues in data collection and processing. *Also see* **GCP, Audit**, and **Research governance**.

ChatGPT : *See* **Generative AI**.

Cherry-picking: Reporting particular data and results while omitting others. *Also see* **p-hacking**.

Chief investigator : An investigator who is responsible for the conduct of the whole trial throughout its lifecycle from inception to post-publication. *See* **Principal investigator**.

Citizen science : An open science initiative encouraging public and consumer involvement in scientific research with citizens actively making intellectual contributions, not simply participating passively as research subjects. Thus citizen science is research being carried out with or by citizens rather than it being undertaken about or for them. *Also see* **Open science** and **Patient and public involvement**.

Clinical investigator : Healthcare professionals who execute trials in clinical practice according to the approved protocol. Where a trial site has many clinical investigators, one of them serves as the site principal investigator. In some circumstances, clinical investigator may also be one of the principal investigators. *Also see* **Site principal investigator, Principal investigator**, and **Trialist**.

Clinical practice guideline : Statements that aim to assist practitioners and patients in making decisions about specific clinical situations. They often, but not always, deploy evidence syntheses, e.g., in the form of systematic reviews. *Also see* **RIGHT** and **AGREE II**.

Clinical trial : In the biomedical literature it is a loosely defined term generally meaning a study of the effects of healthcare interventions. The term encompasses a range of study designs including large randomized clinical trials of patients at one end and uncontrolled observations of a few healthy volunteers at the other. Clinical trials are conducted in phases for drug regulatory approval. The details of non-randomized clinical trials are outside the scope of this book. In this book the term trial refers specifically to randomized clinical trials. *Also see* **Phase I–IV clinical trials, Trial, Efficacy,** and **Effectiveness.**

CoARA : The Coalition for Advancing Research Assessment commits to reviewing and developing criteria, tools and processes for assessing research organizations, and to abandoning inappropriate uses of quantitative journal- and publication-based metrics (coara.eu). *Also see* **Publish or perish, SCOPE,** and **DORA.**

Coercion authorship : *See* **Guest authorship.**

Coercive citation practices : Peer reviews and journals may coerce authors into including references to their own papers during manuscript revisions to boost their own citation metrics such as *h*-index and impact factor. *Also see* ***h*(Hirsh)–index, Impact factor, Inadequate citation practices,** and **Publication process manipulation.**

Collaboration authorship : Individuals collaborating to include each other on a series of papers without making substantial contribution to all the papers in the series. *Also see* **Convenience authorship, Authorship abuse, Ghost authorship, Orphan authorship,** and **Unethical authorship.**

Complainant : *See* **Whistleblower.**

Complaint : A written notification of a suspected case of research misconduct or questionable research practice made to a body that has an investigative role, e.g., institution, funder, journal, professional regulator, etc. The notification is sometimes also known as a formal complaint. Complaints can be lodged anonymously. *Also see* **GCP, Questionable research practice, Research integrity,** and **Research misconduct.**

Composite outcome : Combination of two or more component outcomes into a composite. Participants may be said to have experienced the composite outcome when they suffer any one of the components. Composite outcomes are used when individual core outcomes have low event rates. In this situation, composite outcomes can be constructed to help reduce the sample size or the follow-up period or both to make for a feasible trial. The components of the composite outcome should be of a similar level of patient-relevance, similar frequency of occurrence over the follow-up period and similar in response to the intervention. Otherwise, it may be difficult to interpret effects comparing composite outcomes between groups. *Also see* **Outcome, Surrogate outcome, Core outcomes set,** and **Effect.**

Conceptualization : One of 14 terms in the contributor roles taxonomy that gives credit for research idea formulation or development of research goals, aims, objectives, hypothesis, etc. *Also see* **CRediT.**

Confidence interval : The range within which the value of a measurement, e.g., the effect of an intervention, is expected to lie in a population with a given degree of certainty. Confidence intervals represent the distribution probability of random errors, but not of systematic errors (bias). Conventionally, 95% confidence intervals are used. The width of the confidence interval is related to the sample size and the numbers with outcome within the trial groups. *Also see* **Frequentist statistical methods**, **Precision of effect**, and **Random error.**

Confidentiality :   Keeping disclosed information private. In research misconduct investigations, organizations and individuals involved have an obligation to keep the information shared with them under their own control. Disclosure is made only on a need-to-know basis. In some circumstances, disclosure may be required by the law. *Also see* **Confidentiality breach** and **Defamation**.

Confidentiality breach :   A form of research misconduct whereby organizations and individuals disclose to others information shared with them in confidence. Explicit prior permission is required from the owner of the information for proper disclosure. *Also see* **Confidentiality**, **Defamation**, and **Research misconduct**.

Confirmatory trial :   A randomized clinical trial that gathers effectiveness evidence in a large sample of human participants with the disease or condition targeted by the intervention. *Also see* **Phase III clinical trial**, **Trial**, **Effectiveness**, and **Pilot trial**.

Conflicts of interest :   Potential or perceived compromise in the objectivity or judgement of anyone involved in research and publication (an author, editor, peer reviewer, ethics committee member, funding panel member, trial oversight committee member, research misconduct investigation committee member, etc.) due to financial or personal (non-financial) interests. Financial interests include anything where payment is involved, e.g., employment, research and project funding, consultancies, ownership of stock and shares or options, honoraria, patents, paid expert testimony, etc. A distinction is made between funding directly supporting a particular research project and that obtained for other projects; the former does not form a conflict of interest for that particular research project. Personal interests that could influence objectivity or judgment are harder to identify and may include academic rivalries, intellectual passions, religious or political beliefs, etc. The existence of a conflict of interest does not automatically mean that there is or has been a compromise; transparency requires declaration. Lack of declaration of conflicts of interests is research misconduct. ICMJE provides a proforma for this declaration (icmje.org/disclosure-of-interest). *Also see* **Funding disclosure** and **Research misconduct**.

Confounding :   A situation in trials where the effect of the trial intervention is distorted due to the association of the outcome with another factor, the confounding variable, which can prevent or cause the outcome independent of the intervention. It occurs when groups being compared are different with respect to important factors other than the interventions under investigation. Adjustment for confounding requires stratified or multivariable analysis. *Also see* **Randomization** and **Multivariable analysis**.

Consensus :   A method to determine the extent to which stakeholders whether patients or practitioners agree about a given issue. Questionnaire surveys are frequently used to measure consensus but a range of other methods also exist. Setting priorities and determining the importance of outcomes may deploy consensus methods. *Also see* **Focus group**.

CONSORT :   A group of reporting guidelines checklists for the minimum content of manuscripts of trials of different designs (Consolidated Standards of Reporting Trials, consort
-statement.org). *Also see* **SPIRIT**, **SAGER**, and **STROBE**.

Continuous data :   Measurement on a continuous scale such as height, weight, blood pressure, etc. For continuous data, the effect is often expressed in terms of mean difference. *Also
see* **Binary data**.

Contributor :   *See* **Trialist**.

Control event rate (CER) :   The proportion of participants in the control group in whom an
outcome is observed, in a defined time period of follow-up.

Convenience authorship :   Maximizing the number of publications by mutual reciprocity between authors without regard for contribution. *Also see* **Collaboration authorship, Authorship abuse, Ghost authorship, Orphan authorship**, and **Unethical authorship**.

COPE :   Committee on Publication Ethics. Among other things, it issues guidance to journals
on handling allegations of research misconduct (publicationethics.org). *Also see* **Journal,
ICMJE**, and **WAME.**

Core outcomes set :   A minimum set of critical and important outcomes on which there is
consensus that they directly measure what is clinically relevant. Systematic reviews are used to
create a long list of outcomes which is then reduced to a core outcomes set through consensus
surveys collating evaluations of patients and practitioners. *Also see* **Outcome** and **Consensus**.

Corresponding author :   An author of a trial report who is responsible for communication
with the journal during the manuscript submission, its peer review, revisions and publications,
and subsequently in any post-publication correspondence.

Corrigendum :   The publication of a correction notice concerning a paper's version of record.
A corrigendum refers to the correction of an authors' error(s) in the research work where
some elements of the paper may be affected but its research integrity and main findings
remain intact. A corrigendum requires approval by all authors and may be subject to editorial
and peer review assessment. *Also see* **Version of record, Retraction, Research misconduct**,
and **Erratum**.

CRediT :   Contributor Roles Taxonomy is a system for classifying the roles played by individual
authors and those acknowledged in a trial publication. It recognizes and defines the following contributions (in alphabetical order): conceptualization, data curation, formal analysis,
funding acquisition, investigation, methodology, project administration, resources, review and
editing of draft, software, supervision, validation, visualization, and writing of original draft
(DOI: 10.1087/20150211). *Also see* individual role definitions.

Critical appraisal :   Transparent evaluation of medical literature, whether primary studies such
as trials or their systematic reviews, for their integrity, validity, precision and usefulness. Appraisal concerning validity evaluates study quality or risk of bias. Traditionally evidence-based
medicine restricts appraisal to evaluating internal validity, precision and applicability (external
validity). *Also see* **Research integrity, Risk of bias, Precision**, and **External validity**.

Data and Safety Monitoring Board or DSMB :   *See* **Data Monitoring Committee (DMC)**.

Data Curation :   One of 14 terms in the contributor roles taxonomy that gives credit for management activities to annotate (produce metadata necessary for interpreting the data itself) and maintain research data for initial use and later reuse. *Also see* **CRediT**.

Data Monitoring Committee (DMC) :   The DMC, also known as Data and Safety Monitoring Board or DSMB, is composed of independent experts. It reports to the Trial Steering Committee (TSC) making recommendations regarding trial continuation, modification or termination. It may confidentially review the accumulating unblinded trial data (interim analysis) during the course of the trial, and this may have statistical implications for the final data analysis. The TSC and the trial management group may be invited to an open part of the DMC meeting, but not the confidential review. The details of statistical issues in data monitoring and confidential interim analysis are outside the scope of this book (Data Monitoring Committees: Lessons, Ethics and Statistics or DAMOCLES report, DOI: 10.3310/hta9070). *Also see* **Non-maleficence**, **Trial steering committee**, **Trial management group**, **Site principal investigator**, and **Chief investigator**.

Data sharing :   The data transparency principle that trials should share the deidentified or anonymized dataset to allow independent replication of the reported results as well as to derive other benefits such as contribution to evidence syntheses with individual participant data (IPD) meta-analyses and performance of secondary analyses. This requires sharing the full analyzable dataset derived from the raw data accompanied by metadata describing the dataset. It should be prepared deidentified in compliance with privacy laws and sited in a secure repository. *Also see* **FAIR** and **Individual participant data (IPD) meta-analyses**.

Data sleuthing :   Post-publication investigation of possible research misconduct and questionable research practices by volunteer researchers. Data sleuths tend to report their findings via blogging, social media, and academic online platforms such as PubPeer (pubpeer.com). Sleuthing involves use of validated (e.g., digital image forensics, plagiarism checks) as well as so far unvalidated instruments to signpost the possibility of research integrity flaws. *Also see* **Peer review**, **Whistleblower**, **Questionable research practice**, **Research integrity**, and **Research misconduct**.

Defamation :   Discrediting someone or harming their reputation through a false verbal, video (slander) or written (libel) communication. Confidentiality is required in whistleblowing and research misconduct investigations to help protect against causing defamation. *Also see* **Whistleblower** and **Confidentiality**.

DELTA :   A checklist for reporting the sample size calculation in a randomised clinical trial (Difference ELicitation in TriAls, DOI: 10.1136/bmj.k3750). *Also see* **Power (statistical)**.

Discrimination :   The result of applying policies and practices to some but not to others depending on their protected characteristics, i.e., gender, race, religion, disability, sexual orientation, age, etc. *Also see* **Equality and diversity**, **Orphan authorship**, and **Ethics dumping**.

DOAJ :   Directory of Open Access Journals is a worldwide index of open access journals (doaj.org). *Also see* **Journal**, **Open access publication**, and **OASPA**.

DORA :   The Declaration on Research Assessment (DORA) recognizes the need to improve how researchers and their outputs are evaluated, eliminating the use of journal-based metrics, and instead assessing research on its own merits, in funding, appointment, and promotion considerations (sfdora.org/read). *Also see* **Publish or perish**, **SCOPE**, and **CoARA**.

Double jeopardy in research misconduct investigation :   Authors should be protected from being subjected to investigation twice for the same misconduct allegation or complaint when a previous investigation has found that there is no case to answer.

Duplication :   *See* **Plagiarism.**

Effect (effect measure, treatment effect, estimate of effect, effect size) :   Effect is the observed association between interventions and outcomes or a statistic to summarize the direction and magnitude of the observed association. The statistic could be a relative risk, odds ratio, risk difference, or number needed to treat for binary data; a mean difference, or standardized mean difference for continuous data; or a hazard ratio for survival data. The effect has a point estimate and a confidence interval. In evidence syntheses, the term individual effect is often used to describe effects observed in individual trials included in the systematic review and the term summary effect is used to describe the effect generated by pooling the individual effects in a meta-analysis. *Also see* **Confidence interval**, **Point estimate**, **p-value**, and **Precision**.

Effectiveness :   The extent to which an intervention produces a beneficial effect in the routine setting. Unlike efficacy, it seeks to address the question: Does an intervention work under ordinary day-to-day circumstances? Effectiveness trials tend to be pragmatic with adequate sample sizes, intention-to-treat analyses and an emphasis on generalizability when defining participant eligibility criteria. Sometimes a distinction is made between effectiveness in patients and effectiveness in practice. The term efficacy may sometimes be used to describe effectiveness in patients and the term theoretical efficacy may be used for effects observed in ideal, highly controlled, settings. *Also see* **Usefulness of trials**, **Phase III clinical trial**, **Pragmatic trial**, and **Efficacy.**

Efficacy :   The extent to which an intervention can produce a beneficial effect in an ideal, highly controlled, setting. Sometimes the term theoretical efficacy is used to capture this concept; in this context, the term efficacy may be used to describe effectiveness in patients. *Also see* **Phase II clinical trial** and **Effectiveness**.

Eligibility criteria :   The participant inclusion and exclusion criteria. Eligible, consenting participants are randomized and followed up until outcome data are collected. *Also see* **Participants**.

Equality and diversity :   Equality implies that people should not be disadvantaged because of differences in their gender, race, religion, disability, sexual orientation, minority group membership, age, etc. (also known as protected characteristics). Diversity recognizes the differences. *Also see* **Discrimination** and **Ethics dumping**.

EQUATOR :   A network established for improving health research reporting (Enhancing the QUAlity and Transparency Of health Research, equator-network.org). *Also see* **SPIRIT**, **CONSORT**, **SAGER**, and **STROBE**.

Equipoise :   A state of uncertainty about the effect of an intervention affecting its use in practice. The term clinical equipoise is used to refer to this uncertainty at the level of the professional community, not the individual practitioner. Variations in practice and clinical practice guideline recommendations offer evidence of this uncertainty. *Also see* **Consensus**.

Erratum :   The publication of a correction notice concerning a paper's version of record. The term erratum refers to the correction of a journal's error in the publishing process. A minor publishing error may be corrected by the journal without any author input, but authors should be notified. *Also see* **Version of record**, **Retraction**, **Corrigendum**, and **Research misconduct**.

Ethics :   Decision-making guided by moral values that distinguish between right and wrong. The fundamental ethical principles are autonomy (self-determination), beneficence (promote wellbeing), non-maleficence (do no harm), and justice (fairness). *Also see* **Moral values** and **Human research ethics committee**.

Ethics dumping :   Exploitative practices in research partnerships involving high-income and lower-income settings whereby the high-income partner takes advantage of the imbalances of power, resources and knowledge. The global code of conduct for equitable research partnerships, also known as the TRUST code, stipulates the inclusion of lower-income settings throughout the research and publication process (globalcodeofconduct.org). *Also see* **Justice**, **Discrimination**, **Orphan authorship**, **Power**, and **Equality and diversity**.

Evidence synthesis :   A systematic approach to collating relevant evidence to address a research question. The questions may be narrow or broad. Typical evidence syntheses are systematic reviews and meta-analyses of narrow questions, e.g., determining the effect of a single intervention. Broad questions, e.g., comparison of multiple interventions for the same condition, are addressed in umbrella reviews, network meta-analyses and clinical practice guidelines. Scoping and mapping reviews tend to be without clear research questions and they help to define a topic and to identify research gaps. *Also see* **Review**, **Systematic review**, **Meta-analysis**, **Umbrella review**, **Network meta-analysis**, **Clinical practice guideline**, **Scoping review**, **Mapping review**, **Research gap**, and **PROSPERO**.

Evidence-based medicine (EBM) :   Also known as evidence-based practice (EBP), it is the conscientious, explicit and judicious use of current best research evidence in making healthcare decisions. It involves the process of systematically finding, appraising and using contemporaneous research findings as the basis for clinical decisions. Another related term, evidence-based healthcare, extends EBM to all professions associated with healthcare, including purchasing and management. Trustworthy randomized clinical trials and their evidence syntheses provide strong evidence to support EBM. *Also see* **Randomized clinical trials** and **Systematic reviews**.

Explanatory trial :   A randomized trial conducted under ideal, highly controlled, conditions to gather preliminary evidence on the efficacy and safety of an intervention among carefully selected participants (limiting applicability). *Also see* **Phase II clinical trial**, **Trial**, **Pilot trial**, **Efficacy**, and **Research translation**.

Expression of concern :   A note published by a journal to inform readers of there being possibility of a concern about the integrity of a paper. *Also see* **Retraction**, **Research misconduct**, and **Questionable research practices**.

External validity :   *See* **Applicability**.

Fabrication :   Making up data or results for using them as if they were genuine. It is one of the three cardinal sins listed in the FFP definition of research misconduct. *Also see* **FFP**, **Questionable research practices**, and **Research misconduct**.

FAIR :   Data sharing acronym abbreviating that data should be Findable, Accessible, Interoperable and Reusable (DOI: 10.1038/sdata.2016.18). *Also see* **Data sharing**.

Fake peer review :   A form of publication process manipulation whereby fabricated contact details are supplied in the preferred peer reviewers list to journals at the time of manuscript submission and then positive reviews are supplied from these fabricated addresses. *Also see* **Publication process manipulation**.

Falsification :   Manipulating or omitting research data or results and using them as if they were genuine. For example, a data subset that does not support a desired conclusion may be omitted. Image manipulation is also a form of falsification. It is one of the three cardinal sins listed in the FFP definition of research misconduct. *Also see* **FFP**, **Questionable research practices**, and **Research misconduct**.

Feasibility study :   Preliminary studies, usually without randomization, carried out during the design stage or planning of a large randomized clinical trial. They do not address effectiveness. *Also see* **Phase II clinical trial**, **Trial**, **Efficacy**, and **Pilot trial**.

FFP :   Fabrication, Falsification and Plagiarism, regarded as the unholy trinity or the cardinal sins that define research misconduct. There are many other practices included in the definition of research misconduct depending on the jurisdiction. *Also see* **Questionable research practices** and **Research misconduct**.

File drawer problem :   The tendency of journals to publish positive instead of negative results regardless of trial integrity and quality. This leaves statistically non-significant trials in the researchers' file drawers. *Also see* **Publication bias** and **p-hacking**.

Fishing expedition :   Performing multiple tests in a dataset without an *a priori* hypothesis and statistical analysis plan. For instance, repeatedly categorizing continuous variables without justification until a particular cut-off gives a statistically significant result. *Also see* **p-hacking**, **Selective outcome reporting**, and **Statistical analysis plan**.

Focus group :   A qualitative research method. The collection of qualitative data using a group interview on a topic. Usually, 6-12 participants are involved, and they can be used to gauge issues of importance. Setting priorities and determining the importance of outcomes may deploy focus groups. *Also see* **Consensus**.

Forensic statistical analysis :   An analysis undertaken in the investigation of alleged research misconduct. Using the dataset of the trial that is the subject of the allegation forensic statistics are applied to check the raw data file or the statistical analysis file derived from the raw dataset or the statistical analyses reported, etc. The raw data examination may include checks for data ranges, distributions, digit preference, etc. There may be a need to revert to the original case report forms to ensure that the dataset includes the data actually collected. *Also see* **Case report form** and **Research misconduct**.

Forest plot : A graphical display of individual trial effects with 95% confidence intervals in a systematic review along with the summary effect, if meta-analysis is used. It shows at a glance the variation in individual effects from trial to trial (heterogeneity). *Also see* **Meta-analysis** and **Heterogeneity**.

Formal analysis : One of 14 terms in the contributor roles taxonomy that gives credit for the application of statistical, mathematical, computational or other formal techniques to analyze or synthesize trial data. *Also see* **CRediT**.

Fraud : Any intentional act of deception in research violating research integrity. *Also see* **Research misconduct**.

Freedom of Information : The right of individuals to have access to information that pertains to them.

Frequentist statistical methods : These are the most commonly used methods in trials. The hypothesis formulated typically states that there is no difference in outcomes between the intervention and control groups, i.e., the new intervention does not work (null hypothesis). Using the outcome data collected per group, the null hypothesis is tested at a prespecified probability threshold (usually $p=0.05$). Rejection of the null hypothesis at this threshold implies that there is a difference in outcomes between the intervention group compared to control. The effect estimated, e.g., relative risk of the outcome in the intervention group *versus* control, is a point estimate which comes with a range of possible effects contained within its 95% confidence interval. Bayesian methods are not within the scope of this book. *Also see* **Effect, p-value, Power (statistical)**, and **Confidence interval**.

Funder : An organization that provides funding for undertaking a trial. The funders may be governmental agencies, philanthropists, research charities, industry (e.g., pharmaceutical and medical device companies), etc. Funders may provide monies through grants or donations given to institutions administered through contractual agreements. The main funder has a role in scientific quality assurance and securing value for money. *Also see* **Funding disclosure, Funding acquisition, Journal**, and **Institution**.

Funding acquisition : One of 14 terms in the contributor roles taxonomy that gives credit for acquisition of financial support for the trial leading to this publication. *Also see* **CRediT** and **Funding disclosure**.

Funding disclosure : This section of the protocol, article, conference abstract, etc. describes the funding directly supporting the trial. In article submission, this disclosure is usually added in the journal's online portal. It should include the specific grant numbers and full names of funders. Funders themselves may stipulate how their support should be stated. The disclosure must be specific to the trial. Beware that omitting a funder, even if in error, may be perceived as an attempt to hide the support provided. The manuscript should state if the funder played any role in the trial design, conduct, analysis and reporting. This section is not for declaring conflicts of interests. *Also see* **Conflict of interest**, **Funder**, **Funding acquisition**, and **Research misconduct**.

Funnel plot :   A scatter plot of effects in individual trials included in a systematic review against some measure of trial precision, e.g., trial size, inverse of variance, etc. It is used in the exploration of the risk of publication and related biases. Funnel asymmetry suggests the possibility of such biases. *Also see* **Publication bias** and **Variance**.

GCP :   Good clinical practice in human clinical trials or GCP is a set of internationally recognized ethical and professional standards for the design, conduct, recording, analysis and reporting of human clinical trials. In some jurisdictions, trialists are required to have GCP certification updated every two years. *Also see* **Whistleblower**, **Ethics**, and **Human research ethics committee**.

Generalizability :   *See* **Applicability**.

Generative artificial intelligence (AI) :   Artificial Intelligence or AI developments within computer sciences, e.g., ChatGPT or Generative Pretrained Transformer, based on large language models. It goes a step further than traditional AI in that it generates or produces new content such as text, images, etc. It can be deployed in manuscript writing, peer review and editing amongst many other possibilities. Regarding its use transparency is required in the publication process. *Also see* **Artificial intelligence (AI)**.

Ghost authorship :   Purposefully not listing as co-author someone who has made substantial contributions, e.g., to avoid revealing the industry that initiated the trial to make it look like an academic investigator-led project. The unnamed individual may have merited authorship but is not listed as author. This is not to be confused with professional services sought, e.g., in preparing the manuscript for publication, which are usually but not always acknowledged. *Also see* **Authorship abuse**, **Guest authorship**, **Orphan authorship**, **GPP**, and **Unethical authorship**.

Gift authorship :   *See* **Guest authorship**.

Good Research Practice :   *See* **GCP**.

Good Scientific Practice :   *See* **GCP**.

GPP :   Good Publication Practice (GPP) provides guidance on professional medical writing for the publication of commercially sponsored biomedical research be it in the form of manuscripts, conference abstracts or posters, etc. (DOI: 10.7326/M15-0288).

GRADE :   The Grading of Recommendations Assessment, Development and Evaluation (GRADE) working group is an informal collaboration that aims to develop a comprehensive methodology for assessing the strength of the evidence collated in evidence syntheses and for generating recommendations from evidence in clinical practice guidelines (gradeworkinggroup.org). *Also see* **Strength of evidence**.

GRIPP :   A reporting checklist for patient, carer and public involvement in healthcare research (Guidance for Reporting Involvement of Patients and the Public; DOI: 10.1136/bmj.j3453). *Also see* **SPIRIT, CONSORT, SAGER,** and **EQUATOR.**

Guest authorship :   Listing those people as co-authors who have not made substantial contributions. Synonyms include courtesy, gift and honorary authorship. Gift authorship is often offered or sought in the context of mentorship or as a goodwill gesture in advance of a future research collaboration. Coercion authorship involves bullying the research team into accepting them as a guest author. *Also see.* **Authorship abuse, Ghost authorship, Orphan authorship,** and **Unethical authorship.**

Harking: Related to cherry-picking, fishing expedition and p-hacking, this term refers to hypothesizing with the benefit of hindsight, i.e., after the results of multiple tests in a dataset are known. *Also see* **p-hacking.**

Heterogeneity/homogeneity :   The degree to which the individual trial effects in an evidence synthesis are similar (homogeneity) or different (heterogeneity). This may be observed graphically by examining the variation in individual effects (both point estimates and confidence intervals) in a Forest plot. Quantitatively, statistical tests of heterogeneity/homogeneity may be used to determine if the observed variation in effects is greater than that expected due to the play of chance alone. I^2 statistic provides an assessment of heterogeneity ranging from 0% to 100%, giving the percentage of total variation across trials. For making a judgement about reasons behind heterogeneity, one might look at the differences between participants, interventions, outcomes, quality and integrity of trials, deploying meta-regression and sub-group analyses. *Also see* **Forest plot, Meta-regression,** and **Subgroup analysis.**

Highly prolific authorship :   Defined as authors who publish one full paper every five days (more than 72 full papers annually). It may be achieved without meeting authorship criteria, particularly the criterion concerning approval of the manuscript (DOI: 10.1038/d41586-018-06185-8). In this case, it may become a form of guest authorship. *Also see* **Authorship abuse, Guest authorship,** and **Invented authorship.**

***h*(Hirsh)-index :**   A popular statistic to measure scientific output taking account of citations. It is frequently used by institutions in appointments, appraisals and promotions of academic staff and by funders in research grant assessments and awards. For a researcher it is calculated by placing papers (co-)authored by them in rank order of citations (including self-citation) and the value *h* is the number of the rank that is the same as the number of citations. So, an *h*-index of 5 means that the author has 5 published papers that have been cited 5 times or more. Authors may, e.g., through a combination of collaboration authorship, guest authorship, coercive citation practices and gratuitous citations (influencing colleagues to cite them), be able to manipulate this index. It appears that the *h*-index calculation makes no adjustments for article retraction. Journals may also be evaluated using the *h*-index in addition to the impact factor. Coercive citation practices may be deployed by peer reviewers and journals to manipulate these indices. *Also see* **Coercive citation practices, Inadequate citation practices,** and **Publication process manipulation.**

Homogeneity :   *See* **Heterogeneity.**

Human research ethics committee :   Known also by acronyms like REC (Research Ethics Committee) or IRB (Institutional Review Board), these committees are set up under national research regulatory laws. Their membership, including lay members, should have the expertise required to assess the ethical issues in trials. They are tasked principally with the responsibility of giving formal approval to a trial proposal and monitoring the ethical conduct of the trials approved (in some settings, the compliance monitoring role may be undertaken by research governance offices set up by institutions). They may also engage in the education and training of researchers. Note that human research ethics committees are different to ethics committees in hospitals and clinics that address questions related to clinical care. *Also see* **Ethics** and **Research governance**.

ICMJE :   International Committee of Medical Journal Editors. Among other things, it defines the criteria for authorship and gives guidance on the registration of clinical trials (icmje.org). *Also see* **WAME** and **COPE**.

Impact factor (Journal impact factor) :   A popular statistic for ranking journals in order of perceived importance. It is calculated as the mean number of citations per article in a year taking as denominator the total number of citable articles published in the previous two years in a given journal. *Trials*, an open-access journal that charges article processing fees and covers all aspects of randomized clinical trials in healthcare, had a 2022 impact factor of 2.5, i.e., the citable articles it published in 2020 and 2021 were cited on average 2.5 times in 2022 (including self-citation). There are variations on this approach deployed to create different indices for journals. Coercive citation practices may be deployed by journals to manipulate these indices. There appears to be a correlation between journal impact factors and article retraction rates. *Also see* **Coercive citation practices**, **Inadequate citation practices**, and **Publication process manipulation**.

Inadequate citation practices :   Erroneous citations in published articles. These may include unnecessary self-citation as well as citations of works of others that are inappropriate, misleading, missing, inaccurate, etc. Authors should only cite after reading the full text and without any coercion or pressure. *Also see* **Questionable research practices** and **Coercive citation practices**.

Individual participant data (IPD) meta-analysis :   A meta-analysis that uses participant-level data collected in the included trials to produce a summary result. Data sharing makes IPD meta-analysis possible. *Also see* **Meta-analysis** and **Data sharing**.

Inspection :   An audit conducted by an external legally competent authority that has serious implications for the trialists and their institutions in case of a finding of non-compliance with professional standards such as Good Clinical Practice in human clinical trials (GCP). *Also see* **Audit**, **GCP**, **Ethics**, and **Research governance**.

Institution :   A clinical academic organization, e.g., a university or a hospital, that employs trialists. The institution's role covers the lifecycle of a trial leading up to its publication and it focuses on research ethics and governance; journals focus on communication. Funders offer institutions monies to support trials under contractual agreements. Institutions tend to have their own research integrity policies and misconduct investigation procedures, which may operate under the umbrella of national research integrity laws in some countries. *Also see* **Research governance, Ethics, Sponsor, Journal,** and **Funder**.

Institutional Review Board (IRB) : *See* **Human Research Ethics Committee**.

Instrument : A systematic approach to measurement for accurately quantifying and categorizing observations in order to attribute meaning. Checklists used for review quality assessment, e.g., AMSTAR, ROBIS, etc., are validated measurement instruments.

Intellectual honesty : An honest attitude in the pursuit of truth. In research, this may be demonstrated through the acknowledgement of original sources for the ideas used to generate the hypotheses tested, the presentation of facts in an unbiased manner devoid of spin that gives an unjustifiable positive impression in manuscripts, the avoidance of plagiarism, etc. Note that honest errors do not constitute intellectual dishonesty or research misconduct. *Also see* **Scientific virtue, Research integrity,** and **Research misconduct**.

Intention-to-treat (ITT) analysis : A statistical analysis where participants are analyzed according to their initial group allocation, independent of whether they dropped out or not, fully complied with the intervention or not, or crossed over and received alternative interventions. A true ITT analysis includes an outcome (whether observed or estimated) for all participants. *Also see* **Effectiveness, Per-protocol analysis, Attrition bias,** and **Sensitivity analysis**.

Internal validity : *See* **Validity**.

Intervention : A therapeutic or preventative regimen, e.g., a drug, an operative procedure, a dietary supplement, an educational leaflet, a test (followed by a treatment), a mobile health application, etc. undertaken with the aim of improving health outcomes. In a randomized trial, the effect of an intervention is the comparison of outcomes between two groups, one with the intervention and the other without, e.g., placebo, no intervention, standard of care or another control intervention. *Also see* **TIDieR**.

Intervention event rate (IER) : The proportion of participants in the intervention group in whom an outcome is observed, in a specified time period of follow-up. *Also see* **Control event rate**.

Invented Authorship : Naming as co-author a fictitious person or, a colleague or a stranger without their permission. *Also see* **Authorship abuse, Guest authorship, Ghost authorship,** and **Unethical authorship**.

Inverse of variance : *See* **Variance**.

Investigation : One of 14 terms in the contributor roles taxonomy that gives credit for a contributor role in authorship defined as conducting the trial according to its approved protocol including data collection. *Also see* **CRediT**.

Journal : An establishment composed of editors and other publishing staff who organize peer review of trial manuscripts submitted by authors, and publishes digital or print (paper-based) versions of the accepted scientific papers. Journals operate during the trial lifecycle focusing on the communication of information, e.g., they publish protocols during the early life of a trial and trial findings after the trial is completed. *Also see* **Predatory publishing, Open access publication, DOAJ, WAME, ICMJE,** and **COPE.**

Justice :   The fundamental research ethics principle of fairness. To meet this principle, trials must address a relevant societal priority, its participants ought to come from the same population that is expected to reap the benefits of the findings of the completed trial, exclusion criteria cannot unjustifiably be based on a particular characteristic protected by law, etc. *Also see* **Ethics, Moral values, Equality and diversity,** and **Human research ethics committee.**

Mapping review :   An evidence synthesis of an exploratory nature undertaken to describe or map a research topic. These reviews are helpful in determining gaps in the literature to advance a scientific justification for a new trial. *Also see* **Research gap, Scoping review, Evidence synthesis,** and **Systematic review.**

MARS :   A guideline on Meta-Analytic Reporting Standards (*J Bus Psychol* 2013;**28**:123–143; DOI: 10.1007/s10869-013-9300-2). *Also see* **PRISMA.**

Mean difference :   The difference between the means (i.e., the average values) of two groups of measurements on a continuous scale. *Also see* **Effect** and **Continuous data.**

Measurement bias (detection bias, ascertainment bias) :   Systematic differences between groups in how outcomes are assessed in a trial. Blinding of participants and outcome assessors protects against this bias. *Also see* **Bias.**

Meta-analysis :   A statistical technique for combining (pooling) the results of a number of trials addressing the same research question to produce a summary answer. The large majority of meta-analyses summarize aggregate data reported in the published articles included in a systematic review evaluating the effect of an intervention. *Also see* **Systematic review** and **Individual participant data (IPD) meta-analysis.**

Meta-regression :   A multivariable model with effects of individual trials (usually weighted according to their precision using inverse of variance) as the dependent variable and various trial characteristics, e.g., trial integrity and quality, as independent variables. It searches for the influence of trial characteristics on the size of the individual effects observed in an evidence synthesis. *Also see* **Multivariable analysis.**

Methodology :   One of 14 terms in the contributor roles taxonomy that gives credit for the designing of trial. *Also see* **CRediT.**

Misconduct :   *See* **Research misconduct.**

Moral values :   A set of principles that differentiate right from wrong. *Also see* **Ethics, Principle,** and **Standard.**

Multi-arm multi-stage trial :   *See* **Platform trial.**

Multivariable analysis (multivariable model) :   An analysis that relates some independent or explanatory or predictor variables (X1, X2, ...) to a dependent or outcome variable (Y) through a mathematical model such as $Y = \beta 0 + \beta 1X1 + \beta 2X2 + ...$, where Y is the outcome dependent variable, β0 is the intercept term, and β1, β2, ... are the regression coefficients indicating the impact of the independent variables X1, X2, ... on the dependent variable Y. The coefficient is interpreted as the change in the outcome or dependent variable associated with a one-unit change in the independent variable and provides a measure of association or effect. Multivariable analysis is used to adjust for confounding, e.g., by including confounding factors along with the intervention as the independent variables in the model. This way the effect of intervention on outcome can be estimated while adjusting for the confounding effect of other factors. *Also see* **Confounding**.

Network meta-analysis :   A meta-analytic technique that may be used in umbrella reviews addressing broad questions comparing multiple interventions for the same disease or condition. The term network refers to the direct and indirect comparisons of interventions which become available when all systematic reviews of trials of individual interventions available for the same condition are collated in a single overview. Apart from generating a rank order of the interventions for their effects, such evidence syntheses are useful in identifying research gaps and determining the choice of control groups when planning new trials. *Also see* **Systematic review**, **Umbrella review**, and **Meta-analysis**.

Non-maleficence :   The fundamental research ethics principle that potential risks to trial participants ought to be balanced against the benefits to be gained from undertaking trials. The monitoring of risks to trial participants is a key obligation on part of trialists and institutional research governance offices. Depending on the level of risk, independent data monitoring committees may be required to protect participants. *Also see* **Data monitoring committee**, **Ethics**, **Moral values**, and **Human research ethics committee**.

Null hypothesis :   The hypothesis put forward when carrying out statistical significance tests which states that there is no difference in outcomes between groups in a trial. Statistically, we discover if an intervention has an effect by rejecting the null hypothesis that outcomes do not differ between the intervention and the control group. *Also see* **p-value**.

OASPA :   Open Access Scholarly Publishers Association is a community of organizations engaged in open access publication (oaspa.org). *Also see* **Journal**, **Open access publication**, and **DOAJ**.

Odds :   The ratio of the number of participants with an outcome to the number without the outcome in a group. Thus, if out of 100 participants, 30 experienced an outcome (and 70 did not), the odds would be 30/70 or 0.42. *Also see* **Effect**, **Risk**, and **Odds Ratio**.

Odds ratio :   An effect measure for binary data. It is the ratio of odds of an event or outcome in the intervention group to the odds of an outcome in the control group. An OR of 1 indicates no difference between comparison groups. For undesirable outcomes an OR that is < 1 indicates that the intervention is effective in reducing the odds of that outcome. *Also see* **Relative risk**.

Open access publication :   Open knowledge dissemination via free of cost, immediate availability of research outputs and articles online including journal articles. It comes in many forms. At the top end there is immediate open access to the version of record of the article that comes all singing, all dancing as published formally by the journal (gold open access). The other options include preprints or accepted manuscripts before copy editing self-archived by authors possibly with an embargo period introducing some delay in open access (green open access). The future may see the development of legitimate academic-led publishing initiatives that offer immediate open access totally free (diamond open access). *Also see* **Open science, Version of record, Journal, Predatory publishing, OASPA, and DOAJ.**

Open peer review : An umbrella term for the various options available to make peer review compatible with open science principles, including naming peer reviewers (open identities), publishing peer review reports and authors' responses alongside articles (open reports, ideally with DOI's assigned), enabling wider participation in the review process, e.g., by making preprints immediately available on submission for public comment (open pre-review), etc. *Also see* **Open science, PubPpeer, and Peer review.**

Open research data : Open sharing of research data along with published papers so that data can be reused for example to double-check the statistics reported or to perform individual participant data (IPD) meta-analysis. *Also see* **Open science, Meta-analysis, and Data sharing.**

Open science : An umbrella term covering various initiatives like prospective public research registration, open peer review, open access publications, open research data, citizen science, etc. that encourage sharing, cooperation and knowledge dissemination without restrictions. *Also see* **Research transparency.**

ORCID : A unique digital author identifier (orcid.org).

Orphan authorship : Exploiting power imbalance to exclude someone as a co-author, e.g., trainees or colleagues who left the institution before the research is completed are excluded despite their prior contribution, trainees involved in data collection are not given the opportunity to be involved in the drafting of the manuscript, etc. The gender gap in authorship and low representation of less developed country contributors may be a result of this type of authorship abuse. *Also see* **Authorship abuse, Guest authorship, Ethics dumping, Power, and Unethical authorship.**

Outcome : The changes in health status that arise from the disease or condition targeted by interventions or exposure. The intervention aims to reduce bad outcomes (e.g., mortality in cancer) or increase good outcomes (e.g., pregnancy in infertility). In trials, the outcome data are collected for both intervention and control groups. Subjective outcomes may require the input of an outcome adjudication committee blind to participants' group allocation to reduce the risk of measurement bias. The comparison of outcomes between groups is used to estimate the effect. *Also see* **PICO, Core outcomes set, Surrogate outcome, Composite outcome, Effect, and Outcome adjudication committee.**

Outcome adjudication committee : Outcomes including adverse events may be best adjudicated by independent experts or trialists blind to participants' group allocation. This approach aims to standardize outcome assessment against protocol-specified criteria, minimizing the risk of measurement bias in trials with subjectivity in assessments. *Also see* **Adverse event, Outcome, and Measurement bias.**

Overview :   *See* **Umbrella review**.

p-hacking :   A manipulation of data analysis whereby different statistical tests are repeatedly applied until one of them turns up significant, i.e., the p-value observed crosses the statistical significance threshold (e.g., p<0.05). To avoid this problem trials, an *a priori* statistical analysis plan should pre-specify a single analytic strategy for testing the main hypothesis concerning the primary outcome. *Also see* **p-value**, **Statistical analysis plan**, and **Selective outcome reporting**.

p-value (statistical significance) :   The probability, given a null hypothesis, that the observed effects or more extreme effects in a trial could have occurred due to play of chance (random error). In a trial, it is the probability of finding an effect by chance as unusual as, or more unusual than, the one calculated, given that the null hypothesis is correct. Conventionally, a p-value of < 5% (i.e., p < 0.05) has been regarded as statistically significant. This threshold, however, should never be allowed to become a straitjacket. For instance, when there is a risk of spurious significance, e.g., multiple testing in subgroup analysis, a more stringent threshold (e.g., p < 0.01) may be used. Alternatively, a correction, e.g., Bonferroni, may be used to adjust the p-value when applying multiple statistical tests. When interpreting the significance of effects, p-values should always be used in conjunction with confidence intervals. *Also see* **Frequentists statistical methods** and **Confidence interval**.

Paid authorship :   Buying co-authorship without making a contribution. Paper mills are a market for selling authorship usually of fake papers but there is also a market for buying and selling co-authorship of genuine paper. *Also see* **Paper mills**.

Paper mills :   The business of publishing fake research papers and selling authorship. A group of international stakeholders is developing consensus over how to address the challenge paper mills pose (united2act.org). *Also see* **Unethical publication practices**, **Paid authorship**, and **Publication process manipulation**.

Participants :   Individuals, also known as subjects, who meet the eligibility criteria and give informed consent for taking part in a trial. In randomized clinical trials, participants are patients, not healthy volunteers (exceptions include prevention trials such as vaccine trials). Interventions target the disease or condition participants suffer. It is important to define their characteristics in terms of eligibility criteria when formulating structured research questions for trials. Eligible, consenting participants are randomized and followed up until outcome data are collected. Participation is voluntary and guided by informed consent. There is no obligation to stay within the trial until its completion. Healthcare professionals are responsible for ensuring that patients are not forced to enter into trials. *Also see* **PICO**, **Intervention**, **Outcome**, and **Eligibility criteria**.

Patient and public engagement or involvement (PPE or PPI) :   *See* **Patient, carer and public involvement**.

Patient, carer and public involvement or PPI :   Input of lay members of the public in areas such as trial priority setting, core outcome selection, protocol development, consent procedures, participant recruitment and retention, etc. Not included among the 14 terms in the contributor roles taxonomy, it is a recognized role in a trial publication. *Also see* **CRediT, Citizen science,** and **GRIPP.**

Peer review : Formal evaluation of scientific manuscripts by others working in the same field prior to their publication as definitive articles representing the version of record. Traditionally, peer review is undertaken at the invitation of journal editors with the objective of having the submitted manuscripts assessed for their merit, including amongst other things a filter for research integrity. Pre-review and post-publication peer review are uninvited evaluations. Authors have a duty to respond to all the comments made, whether or not formally invited by the journal. *Also see* **PubPeer** and **Open peer review.**

Per-protocol analysis : An analysis where participants who who dropped out, did not fully comply with or discontinued the intervention, crossed over or received alternative interventions are excluded. This analytic approach pertains to efficacy, not effectiveness trials. *Also see* **Effectiveness, Efficacy Intention-to-treat analysis,** and **Explanatory trial.**

Performance bias : Systematic differences in the care provided to the study subjects other than the interventions being evaluated. Blinding of carers and subjects and standardization of the care plan can protect against this bias. *Also see* **Selection bias.**

Phase I clinical trial : A clinical trial focussing on the safety of an intervention in a few healthy human volunteers. Randomization is not used. *Also see* **Clinical trial.**

Phase II clinical trial : A clinical trial that gathers preliminary evidence on whether an intervention works in human participants. It may or may not involve randomization. The preliminary evidence gathered may be used to help define the intervention better including dose finding (Phase IIa) and to determine its efficacy via a randomized clinical trial in a small number of carefully selected participants with the disease or condition targeted by the intervention (Phase IIb). *Also see* **Clinical trial, Proof-of-concept study, Explanatory trial,** and **Efficacy.**

Phase III clinical trial : A clinical trial that gathers evidence on the effectiveness of an intervention. It involves randomization of a large number of human participants with the disease or condition targeted by the intervention. Prevention trials such as vaccine trials recruit healthy participants. *Also see* **Clinical trial, Effectiveness, Pragmatic clinical trial,** and **Confirmatory trial.**

Phase IV clinical trial : A clinical trial that gathers additional information about an approved drug's safety or optimal use in healthcare practice. *Also see* **Clinical trial.**

PICO : An acronym describing various trial components. P stands for participants, I for intervention, C for comparison and O for outcomes. *Also see* **Participants, Intervention,** and **Outcome.**

Pilot trial : A randomized clinical trial in miniature form to examine the coherence of the various elements of a planned large randomized clinical trial. It is not designed to address effectiveness. It estimates effects imprecisely owing to a small sample size. It primarily serves to examine the practicability of the trial protocol; glitches found can be corrected before proceeding with the large definitive trial. Sometimes pilot trials, known as internal pilots, are undertaken within large trials at their beginning. *Also see* **Phase II clinical trial**, **Trial**, **Efficacy**, and **Feasibility study**.

Plagiarism :   Copying the work of others (text, tables, images, data) and presenting it as if it were own work without proper citation to the original source. Self-plagiarism, auto-plagiarism and recycling are terms used to describe forms of plagiarism where authors copy own works, representing them with minor changes without citation to their own previous publications. Duplication, another synonym, may refer to plagiarism or self-plagiarism. A redundant publication is work multiply published in part or in its entirety (in the same or another language) without justification and without reference to the original source. Depending on the extent of the material copied, the originality of the material copied, and citations to the original source, plagiarism may be classified as questionable research practice or misconduct. Plagiarism checks can be carried out using artificial intelligence and it is a common reason for article retraction. *Also see* **FFP**.

Platform trial :   A randomized, adaptive trial, to assess multiple interventions with the option to continue, add or discontinue trial arms at each stage of statistical analysis according to a pre-specified plan. A multi-arm, multi-stage trial is differentiated from a platform trial by having a fixed end date, but they share the common aim of evaluating all available options for the treatment of a target disease or condition. *Also see* **Clinical trial**, **Pragmatic clinical trial**, and **Confirmatory trial**.

Point estimate of effect :   The value of the effect of a trial intervention among the participant sample. *Also see* **Effect** and **Confidence interval**.

Policy :   A guideline or set of rules of an organization. *Also see* **Procedure** and **Regulation**.

Power :   The ability to influence others. In the healthcare setting, role asymmetry permits healthcare professionals to influence patients. The personal authority healthcare professionals exercise over vulnerable patients can sometimes lead to abuse. It is the responsibility of healthcare professionals to ensure that patients are never forced to enter into trials as participants. Consent for participation should be fully informed and entirely voluntary. In the academic setting, the power imbalance between research colleagues may also be abused in unethical authorship. *Also see* **Participants** and **Authorship abuse**.

Power (statistical) :   The ability to reject the null hypothesis when it is indeed false. Power is related to sample size and the number of outcomes in the comparison groups. The larger the sample size, the more the power, the narrower the confidence interval around the point estimate of the effect of the intervention, and the lower is the risk that a possible effect could be missed due to the play of chance. *Also see* **Confidence interval**, **Random error**, and **DELTA**.

Pragmatic clinical trial :   A randomized clinical trial that gathers evidence on the effectiveness of an intervention in the real-world setting for optimisation of its use in healthcare practice. It involves randomization of a large number of participants with the target condition. For approved drugs, these trials are conducted after market access has been granted. Trial pragmatism features include: participants with eligibility criteria that capture the condition targeted by intervention in the healthcare setting; interventions delivered with the resources, expertise and flexibility of real-world practice; comparators based on alternative treatments available as part of the standard of care; outcomes measured with patient-relevant endpoint; and analyses by intention-to-treat. Some pragmatic studies of correlations of interventions with outcomes may not deploy randomization. *Also see* **Usefulness of trials, Effectiveness, Phase III clinical trial, Trial,** and **Applied research.**

Precision of effect : *See* **Random error.**

Predatory publishing : Open access journals publishing irresponsibly, putting financial interest ahead of the trustworthiness of the research record. *Also see* **Journal, Open access publication, OASPA,** and **DOAJ.**

Preprint : A publicly posted draft version of a scientific manuscript prior to completion of its formal peer review. It is usually simultaneously posted at the first submission of a manuscript to a journal. It offers the opportunity for public comment (pre-review) alongside formal peer review organized by the journal. Preprints are not considered prior publication, so they are not disqualifiers for submission to a journal. Preprints usually have DOI's (digital object identifiers) and can be cited like any other paper. The preprint version is updated with a link to the final published version. *Also see* **Open science, Version of record, Open access,** and **Peer review.**

Principal investigator : A term that varies in its use across countries, academic settings and research cultures. It may be equivalent to a Chief investigator in some settings. In other settings, the principal investigator may be the site principal investigator. *Also see* **Chief investigator** and **Site principal investigator.**

Principle : A moral value and concept, i.e., something that distinguishes between right and wrong, for guiding trialists' behavior. *Also see* **Standard, Ethics** and **Moral values.**

PRISMA : A group of reporting checklists for the minimum content of manuscripts of systematic reviews, meta-analyses and their protocols focusing on evidence syntheses evaluating the effects of interventions using randomized clinical trials (Preferred Reporting Items for Systematic Reviews and Meta-Analyses, prisma-statement.org). Also see **MARS, AGREE II, AMSTAR-2, RIGHT,** and **ROBIS.**

Procedure : Step-by-step instructions for implementing a policy in an organization. *Also see* **Policy** and **Regulation.**

Professional regulatory body : By law, healthcare professionals must be registered with a professional regulatory body to ensure they are fit and licensed to practice. Regulated healthcare professionals are many, including but not limited to biomedical scientists, chiropractors, clinical scientists, dentists, dental nurses and technicians, dietitians, doctors, hearing aid dispensers, midwives, nurses, nursing associates, occupational therapists, operating department practitioners, opticians, osteopaths, paramedics, pharmacists, physiotherapists, radiographers, speech and language therapists, etc. (in alphabetical order). A regulatory body may undertake a fitness-to-practice investigation upon being alerted about a research integrity concern. The term professional regulatory body should not be confused with the term regulator used in this book. The latter is a formal body set up for official approvals of medicines and devices, e.g., European Medicines Agency (EMA). *Also see* **Regulator**.

Professional Societies : *See* **Societies**.

Prognosis : The anticipated outcome in the usual course of a disease or condition. In trials, the term baseline risk is sometimes used to refer to the frequency of outcomes without intervention, e.g., in the control group of participants who may receive no treatment or placebo. It is related to the severity of underlying disease and prognostic features. Good prognosis is associated with low baseline risk while poor prognosis is associated with high baseline risk. Interventions intend to improve the prognosis. In trials, the table of baseline characteristics gives the key prognostic variables of the randomized groups. Randomization with allocation concealment aims to produce groups similar at baseline with respect to prognosis. If the groups are imbalanced for prognostic at baseline, something that may happen due to chance imbalance, the analysis benefits from the incorporation of these variables in the estimation of the effect through multivariable analysis. *Also see* **Target condition**.

Project administration : One of 14 terms in the contributor roles taxonomy that gives credit for the management, coordination planning and execution of a trial. *Also see* **CRediT**.

Proof-of-concept study : A term used to describe a clinical trial conducted as an early translational step to inform "go/no-go" decisions about proceeding further with randomized clinical trials. It does not address effectiveness. *Also see* **Phase II clinical trial**, **Explanatory trial**, **Effectiveness**, and **Research translation**.

Prospective trial registration : Pre-registration of a trial in a publicly available registry before the enrolment of the first participant. *Also see* **PROSPERO**.

PROSPERO : A database for prospectively registering evidence syntheses including systematic reviews and umbrella reviews where there is a health-related outcome. It does not accept scoping reviews (crd.york.ac.uk/prospero).

Publication bias : A bias that arises when the likelihood of publication of a study is related to the significance of its results. For example, a trial may be less likely to be published if it finds an intervention ineffective. In evidence synthesis, if such negative trials go missing the inferences about the value of intervention will become biased. Funnel plots may be used to explore for the risk of publication and related biases.

Publication process manipulation : A form of research misconduct in the publication process. It may involve authors as well as reviewers. Examples include organization of or taking part in fake peer review, unauthorized use of information gained through peer reviewing activities, confidentiality violation through disclosure of peer-reviewed information to others and coercive citation practices. *Also see* **Fake peer review**, **Coercive citation practices**, and **Unethical publishing practices**.

Publish-or-perish : An academic culture in which research organizations value the numbers of papers rather than their integrity, quality or impact. *Also see* **DORA**, **CoARA**, and **SCOPE**.

PubMed : Freely available interface of the general biomedical research database Medline which contains publication records with and without abstracts from 1966 onwards (ncbi .nlm.nih.gov/PubMed). It covers around 5,200 journals, whereas it is estimated that there are 16,000 biomedical journals.

PubPeer : An online platform for post-publication peer review (pubpeer.com). *Also see* **Peer review** and **Open peer review**.

Quality of a trial (methodological quality) : The degree to which a trial has minimized biases. Features related to the design, the conduct and the statistical analysis of the trial can be used to measure quality. This assessment focuses on the validity (internal) of the trials, a methodological element distinct from the assessment of the trial's integrity features which may identify flaws due to research misconduct or questionable research practices. *Also see* **Risk of bias assessment, Validity (internal validity),** and **Bias**.

Quality of an evidence synthesis (methodological quality) : The degree to which an evidence synthesis, e.g., a systematic review or a clinical practice guideline, has minimized biases. Features related to the design, the conduct and the statistical analysis of the evidence synthesis can be used to measure quality. This assessment focuses on the validity (internal) of the evidence synthesis, a methodological element distinct from the assessment of review's integrity features which may identify flaws due to research misconduct or questionable research practices. *Also see* **Risk of bias assessment, Validity (internal validity),** and **Bias**.

Quasi-randomized (quasi-experimental) study : A study where allocation of participants to groups is controlled by the researcher, but the method falls short of genuine randomization (and allocation concealment), e.g., by using date of birth or even-odd days. Such studies suffer all the same methodological biases that are inherent in observational studies. *Also see* **Randomized clinical trial**.

Questionable research practices (QRPs) : Irresponsible research practices that are regarded as unethical or unprofessional but fall short of being included in the definition of research misconduct. There are many QRPs including but not limited to selective outcome reporting, the introduction of spin in the description of research findings, etc. *Also see* **Research misconduct**.

Random error (imprecision or sampling error) : Error due to the play of chance that leads to wide confidence intervals around point estimates of effect. The width of the confidence interval reflects the magnitude of random error or imprecision. Variance, a statistical measure, quantifies imprecision. The inverse of variance is often used to weight trials in statistical syntheses, e.g., in meta-analysis, meta-regression and funnel plot analysis. This weighting makes the individual trial with lower variance (i.e., with greater precision in the estimation of trial effect) to have more importance in the calculation. *Also see* **p-value, Power (statistical), Confidence interval, Meta-analysis, Meta-regression,** and **Funnel plot**.

Randomization (with allocation concealment) : Randomization is the allocation of consenting eligible participants to two or more groups using a chance procedure, such as computer-generated random numbers, to generate a sequence for allocation. It ensures that participants have a prespecified (very often an equal) chance of being allocated one of two or more groups. In this way, the groups are likely to be balanced for known as well as unknown and unmeasured confounding variables. Concealment of the allocation sequence until the time of participant allocation to groups is essential for protection against selection bias. Foreknowledge of group allocation leaves the decision to enrol the participants open to manipulation by clinical investigators and by participants themselves. Allocation concealment is almost always possible even when blinding is not. Randomization alone without conceal-ment does *not* protect against selection bias. *Also see* **Selection bias**.

Randomized clinical trial :   A clinical trial involving random allocation of eligible, consenting human participants to arms or intervention groups and their follow-up to compare group out-comes. The random allocation is kept concealed from both trialists and participants until eligibil-ity assessments have been performed and informed consent has been obtained. This book refers to randomized clinical trials throughout as **Trials**. This type of trial is launched after pre-clinical and proof-of-concept studies have established the underlying mechanisms and the plausibility by which the intervention could have an effect on the target condition and have shown it to be likely safe and tolerable. *Also see* **Clinical trial**, **Trial**, **Randomization**, and **Trialist**.

Real-world data and evidence :   Patient data routinely collected during practice or the delivery of healthcare, e.g., from electronic health records, product or disease registries, health insurance data, etc., Real-world evidence is usually generated using these observational data. Pragmatic clinical trials extend into the real-world space in research translation. *Also see* **Pragmatic clinical trials**, **Applied research**, and **Research translation**.

Real-world evidence synthesis :   The extent to which evidence syntheses of trials can be an-ticipated to produce useful results to directly inform healthcare practice and policy. Umbrella reviews with broad questions covering all the available options for the treatment of a disease or condition have the potential to serve decision-making in the healthcare setting. *Also see* **Umbrella reviews**, **Network meta-analysis**, **Real-world data and evidence**, **Pragmatic clinical trial**, and **Applied research**.

Recklessness :   Indifference or disregard towards the risk of potentially false information being produced from research undertaken without exercising proper care or caution. *Also see* **Research misconduct**.

Redundant publication :   *See* **Plagiarism**.

Regulations :   The directives which an authority creates, maintains and enforces by law. *Also see* **Policy**, **Procedure**, and **Regulator**.

Regulator :   A formal body set up for official approvals of medicines and devices, e.g., Euro-pean Medicines Agency (EMA), US Food and Drug Administration (FDA), UK Medicines and Healthcare products Regulatory Agency (MHRA), etc. *Also see* **Regulations**.

Relative risk (risk ratio, rate ratio) :   An effect measure for binary data. It is the ratio of risk in the intervention group to the risk in the control group. An RR of 1 indicates no difference between comparison groups. For undesirable outcomes an RR that is <1 indicates that the intervention is effective in reducing the risk of that outcome. *Also see* **Risk**, **Odds ratio**, and **Effect**.

Replication :   Repeating a piece of research in order to verify or complement the original results. Replication is a recognized good research practice. Trials may be repeated when the previously evaluated effects of interventions need reconfirmation, e.g., when the applicability of previous trial findings needs reassessment in a different setting or in a different participant group or with some modification to the intervention, etc. Human research ethics committees should determine if replication of a trial is necessary before giving approval. *Also see* **TOP**.

Research Ethics Committee (REC) :   *See* **Human Research Ethics Committee**.

Research culture :   The academic environment comprising of the norms, values, expectations, attitudes and behaviors within research organizations. It strongly influences research integrity. For example, the publish-or-perish culture is believed to be associated with authorship abuse. Academic freedom, collegiality, collaboration, equality and diversity, ethics and professionalism, openness and transparency are all features of the research culture. *Also see* **Publish-or-perish, Equality and diversity, Research integrity, Research transparency,** and **Open science**.

Research gap :   A knowledge gap or the inability to answer a research question due to insufficient evidence. *Also see* **Research need** and **Research priority**.

Research governance :   The system set up by institutions to oversee the conduct of trials under their auspices. Governance approvals for trials and oversight of their compliance with standards are enforced through established institutional research policies and procedures. *Also see* **Human Research Ethics Committee, Sponsor, Research integrity,** and **Research ethics**.

Research integrity :   Undertaking trials in accordance with ethical and professional principles and standards. Integrity failures may result from honest or innocent errors as well as from intentional, knowing or reckless research misconduct. *Also see* **Research misconduct** and **Questionable research practices**.

Research misconduct :   Unethical or unprofessional conduct in research that is intentional, knowing or reckless, i.e., negligent. In some definitions, misconduct is limited to fabrication, falsification or plagiarism (FFP), and in others, unethical authorship or authorship abuse, conflict of interest mismanagement, publication process manipulation, and misconduct related to misconduct investigation procedures, etc. are also included. There are many questionable research practices that do not make it into the definition of misconduct. Honest error is not misconduct. *Also see* **Questionable research practices**.

Research need :   A research gap resulting in an inability to make healthcare decisions among patients, practitioners and policymakers. *Also see* **Research gap**.

Research priority :   The ranking or selection of a few among the many established research gaps and needs to help in resource allocation. *Also see* **Research gap** and **Research need**.

Research translation :   Moving from the bench to the bedside, i.e., from theoretical research knowledge about disease mechanisms gained in the laboratory all the way to its application into routine clinical practice and healthcare decision-making. Clinical trials, particularly randomised clinical trials and their evidence syntheses are key translational steps leading to improved health. *Also see* **Pragmatic clinical trials** and **Real-world data and evidence**.

Research transparency :   Transparency in research includes open science practices such as prospective registration, protocol publication, *a priori* statistical analysis plan, data sharing, timely and complete public reporting, etc. *Also see* **Open science**.

Resources :   One of 14 terms in the contributor roles taxonomy that gives credit for the provision of study materials, computing resources, etc. *Also see* **CRediT**.

Respondent in a research misconduct investigation :   The trialist whose research conduct is the subject of a complaint or is being investigated formally by their employer, funder, journal, regulator or the law court. *Also see* **Complaint**, **Questionable research practice**, **Research integrity**, **Research misconduct**, **Professional regulator**, and **Trialist**.

Responsible research conduct :   Research conduct that is compliant with ethical and professional principles and standards. *Also see* **Research integrity**, **Research misconduct**, and **Questionable research practices**.

Retraction :   Withdrawal or removal of a published paper from the research record because of a variety of reasons including the discovery of a flaw in its integrity, e.g., a post-publication reassessment showing that the data or results reported have major errors. A research misconduct investigation may have established that the paper in question harbored research misconduct or perhaps there was an honest error. Journals publish retraction notices and identify retracted papers in electronic databases with reasons for retraction which are not always clearly stated. In case of honest errors, journals may retract and republish a paper or may publish a corrigendum. *Also see* **Expression of concern**, **Erratum or corrigendum**, **Research misconduct**, and **Questionable research practices**.

Review and editing of draft :   One of 14 terms in the contributor roles taxonomy that gives credit for critical review, commentary or revision of the initial manuscript draft. *Also see* **CRediT**.

Review of reviews :   *See* **Umbrella review**.

RIAT :   An international effort to correct the problem of unpublished and misreported (inaccurate or incomplete) trials (Restoring Invisible and Abandoned Trials, restoringtrials.org). *Also see* **AllTrials**.

RIGHT :   A reporting quality instrument for clinical practice guidelines (Reporting Items for practice Guidelines in HealThcare, www.right-statement.org). *Also see* **AGREE II** and **Clinical practice guidelines**.

Risk (proportion or rate) :   The proportion of subjects in a group who are observed to have an outcome. Thus, if out of 100 subjects, 30 had the outcome, the risk (rate of outcome) would be 30/100 or 0.30. *Also see* **Odds**, **Relative risk**, **Risk difference**, and **Odds ratio**.

Risk of bias assessment :   An assessment that determines the validity (internal) of the results of a study (a trial or an evidence synthesis). Specific checklists or instruments are used to perform these assessments. *Also see* **ROB-2, AMSTAR-2, ROBIS, Validity (internal validity), Quality of a trial,** and **Quality of an evidence synthesis**.

ROB-2 : Version 2 of an instrument for assessing the Risk Of Bias in randomised clinical trials (https://methods.cochrane.org/risk-bias-2).

ROBIS : An instrument for assessing the Risk Of Bias In Systematic reviews (www.bristol.ac.uk/population-health-sciences/projects/robis/robis-tool). *Also see* **AMSTAR-2**.

SAGER : A checklist for gender-sensitive reporting (Sex and Gender Equity in Research, DOI: 10.1186/s41073-016-0007-6). *Also see* **SPIRIT, CONSORT,** and **STROBE**.

Salami publication : Presenting the different results of a single study into multiple publications that could have been more justifiably consolidated into a single paper.

Sample : Participants selected for a trial from a much larger group or population. Sample characteristics have a strong bearing on the applicability of trial findings. *Also see* **Participants, Eligibility criteria,** and **Applicability**.

Scientific virtue : A character trait or a disposition to consistently act in a manner that will best achieve scientific excellence. Intellectual honesty, accountability, meticulousness, transparency and other related virtues are essential to research integrity and responsible research conduct. *Also see* **Intellectual honesty, Research integrity,** and **Research misconduct**.

SCOPE : A framework for evaluating research responsibly produced by INORMS, the International Network of Research Management Societies (Start with what is valued, Context considerations, Options for evaluating, Probe deeply and Evaluate the evaluation; DOI: 10.26188/21919527.v1). *Also see* **Publish or perish, CoARA,** and **DORA**

Scoping review : An evidence synthesis without a clearly formulated question undertaken to clarify key concepts in a research topic. *Also see* **Mapping review, Research gap, Evidence synthesis,** and **Systematic review**.

Selection bias (allocation bias) : Systematic differences in prognosis or therapeutic response at baseline between trial groups. Randomization (with concealed allocation) of a large number of participants protects against this bias. *Also see* **Bias** and **Randomization**.

Selective outcome reporting : A difference in the outcomes reported in a published trial compared to its original ethics committee approved protocol and prospective registration. The prospective registration requirements implemented since 2005 have encouraged reporting of the result for the original primary outcome, even if it shows a statistically non-significant result on trial completion. In the past, if the original primary outcome showed a statistically non-significant result on trial completion, there used to be a tendency to report statistically significant results of non-primary outcomes. There may be an element of p-hacking involved even when the primary outcome cannot be easily changed, and that is why an *a priori* statistical analysis plan is required. *Also see* **p-hacking** and **Prospective trial registration**.

Selective reporting : *See* **Selective outcome reporting**.

Self-plagiarism : *See* **Plagiarism**.

Sensitivity analysis : Repetition of an analysis under different assumptions to examine the impact of these assumptions on the results. In trials, when participants dropout their outcome goes missing. Intention-to-treat analysis requires estimated outcomes for which there are many ways to impute the missing. One method should be specified as the primary analysis and the others as sensitivity analysis. Concerning integrity assessment in systematic reviews, when a trial shows an outlier result, sensitivity analysis may include re-running the meta-analysis without the outlier. *Also see* **Intention-to-treat analysis** and **Withdrawals**.

Site investigator : *See* **Site principal investigator**.

Site principal investigator : The trialist or investigator coordinating all trial affairs in a trial site or center. Not included among the 14 terms in the contributor roles taxonomy, it is a recognized role in a trial publication. *Also see* **Principal investigator**, **CRediT**, and **Trialist**.

Societies : A non-profit organization (body or association) that seeks to further a particular healthcare profession and the interests of their patients. Societies are made up of a membership of healthcare professionals. Societies tend to have an official journal, a committee for developing clinical practice guidelines, an annual conference with posters, oral presentations and workshops, etc. Members of professional societies may participate in planning and conducting clinical trials in their specialty. As professionals, they have a seat on the table in determining priorities alongside other stakeholders such as patients, carers and public representatives. *Also see* **Institution, Funder** and **Journal.**

Software : One of 14 terms in the contributor roles taxonomy that gives credit for programming, software development; designing computer programs; implementation of the computer code and supporting algorithms; etc. *Also see* **CRediT**.

Spin : Exaggerating the implications or importance of research findings in order to increase the likelihood of publication. It is a questionable research practice. *Also see* **Questionable research practice**, **Research integrity**, and **Research misconduct**.

SPIRIT : A group of reporting checklists for the minimum content of protocols of trials of different designs (Standard Protocol Items: Recommendations for Interventional Trials; spirit -statement.org/). *Also see* **CONSORT**, **SAGER**, and **STROBE**.

Sponsor : Clinical trials regulations require that a sponsor makes proper arrangements to initiate and conduct trials. For trialists employed in an academic setting, it is usually their own institution that acts as the sponsor. In commercial trials seeking regulatory approval, the sponsor may be a pharmaceutical company. *Also see* **Institution** and **Regulator**.

Standard : Specification of the behavior that must be adhered to when planning, conducting, analyzing and reporting a trial. *Also see* **Principle**, **Ethics**, and **Moral values**.

Statistical analysis plan : Development of the analysis outlined in a trial registration and protocol into a detailed *a priori* statistical analysis plan of the primary outcome, the secondary outcomes and other variables before the dataset is closed and prepared for formal analysis. The database is locked following the collection of the outcome data from the last recruited participant. Not included among the 14 terms in the contributor roles taxonomy, preparation of the statistical analysis plan should be a recognized role in a trial publication. *Also see* **CRediT**, **P-hacking**, and **Selective outcome reporting**.

STROBE : A group of reporting checklists for the minimum content of manuscripts of observational studies of different designs (STrengthening the Reporting of OBservational studies in Epidemiology, strobe-statement.org). *Also see* **SPIRIT**, **CONSORT**, **SAGER**, and **EQUATOR**.

Subgroup analysis : Analyses carried out in prespecified subgroups, e.g., trial analyses stratified according to differences in participant characteristics to examine if the effect of the intervention varies between the subgroups. *Also see* **Meta-analysis**.

Subjects : *See* **Participants**.

Supervision : One of 14 terms in the contributor roles taxonomy that gives credit for oversight and leadership responsibility for research planning and execution, including mentorship. *Also see* **CRediT**.

Surrogate outcome : A substitute for direct measures of changes in health status. Instead of measuring how patients feel, what their function is, or if they survive, they capture short-term physiological variables (e.g., blood pressure for stroke or HbA1c for diabetic complications) or measures of subclinical disease (e.g., degree of atherosclerosis on coronary angiography for future heart attack). To be valuable, the surrogate must be statistically correlated with the clinically relevant outcome. *Also see* **Core outcomes set**, **Composite Outcome**, **Outcome**, and **Effect**.

Systematic error : *See* **Bias**.

Systematic review : An evidence synthesis type that summarizes the evidence on a clearly formulated question, either narrow or broad, using systematic and explicit methods to identify, select and appraise relevant primary studies, and to extract, collate and report their findings. It may or may not use statistical meta-analysis. *Also see* **Evidence synthesis** and **Meta-analysis**.

Target condition : The disease or condition targeted by the intervention for use in healthcare after trials have evaluated effectiveness. For example, in a vaccine trial the target condition may be otherwise healthy people who need protection from an infectious disease in the future, in cancer chemotherapy the target condition may be the cancer diagnosis and stage, etc. The participant eligibility criteria aim to capture the trial sample with features closely matching the target condition. Note that the term target condition is used differently in test accuracy research. *Also see* **Participants**.

TIDieR : A reporting checklist for the completeness of reporting of interventions (Template for Intervention Description and Replication, tidierguide.org). *Also see* **Intervention**, **CONSORT**, **SAGER**, and **SPIRIT**.

TOP : Guidelines for Transparency and Openness Promotion (TOP) in journal policies and practices (osf.io/ud578). *Also see* **Journal** and **TRUST**.

Transparency in research misconduct investigation : The requirement that steps of a research misconduct investigation are clearly laid out to the respondent trialist who has the right to be informed about the process and the stage of the procedure at any time during the investigation. *Also see* **Respondent**.

Trial :   *See* **Randomized clinical trial** and **Trialist**.

Trial arm :   *See* **Arm**.

Trial management group :   The chief investigator oversees the conduct of the trial undertaken by its approved protocol with a management group comprising of co-investigators and appointed staff, e.g., trial manager, data manager, statistician, trial physicians and nurses, etc. They establish and monitor the recruitment of participants in the trial centers working closely with site principal investigators in multicentre trials. They also supervise data collection, entry and cleaning, and service the various trial committees. They take instructions from the chair of the trial steering committee (TSC) which may be set up to provide independent supervision. *Also see* **Trial steering committee**, **Data monitoring committee**, **Site principal investigator**, and **Chief investigator**.

Trial Steering Committee (TSC) :   The TSC, composed of an independent chair and independent members as well as some of the trialists, is responsible for overall trial supervision. It takes responsibility for the scientific integrity of the trial. Typically, the Data Monitoring Committee (DMC) reports to the TSC and trial management group takes instructions from the chair of the TSC. *Also see* **Non-maleficence**, **Trial management group**, **Data monitoring committee**, **Site principal investigator**, and **Chief investigator**.

Trialist :   An investigator who makes a contribution to a trial and is credited in the authorship or the acknowledgement section of the published article. *Also see* **Trial**, **Authorship**, **CRediT**, **Chief investigator**, and **Site principal investigator**.

TRUST :   Transparency of Research Underpinning Social Intervention Tiers (TRUST) initiative that evaluates the implementation of TOP guidelines in journal policies and procedures (DOI: 10.1186/s41073-021-00112-8). *Also see* **Journal** and **TOP**.

Umbrella review (reviews of reviews, overview) :   A review of systematic reviews on a topic. An umbrella review may address a broad question about the comparison of multiple interventions for the same condition using network meta-analysis. An umbrella review that collates several reviews on a narrow question harmonizes the interpretation across existing narrow systematic reviews. *Also see* **Review**, **Systematic review**, **Meta-analysis**, and **Network meta-analysis**.

Unethical Authorship :   Authorship attribution that is not based strictly on contributions that meet authorship criteria. Authorship abuse occurs in many forms including: when authorship is demanded through coercion, e.g., based on seniority, rather than deserved on account of the contribution made (guest authorship); when someone is excluded from authorship even when they have made creditable contributions (ghost authorship); when someone is included as an author without their permission (invented authorship); when names of original contributors are removed in subsequent publications; when there is manipulation of the sequence of authors, particularly first, last and corresponding author, without justification; etc. *Also see* **Authorship abuse**, **Collaboration authorship**, **Convenience authorship**, **Guest authorship**, **Ghost authorship**, **Orphan authorship**, and **Invented authorship**.

Unethical publication practices : Unethical science publishing whereby (predatory) journals take financial advantage of the pressure to publish or perish on researchers. *Also see* **Publish or perish, Publication process manipulation,** and **Paper mill.**

Usefulness of trials : A multidimensional concept, differentiating between basic and applied research, evaluating integrity, research priority, pragmatism, validity, precision, etc. The usefulness concept can be extended to evidence syntheses. *Also see* **Applied research, Real-world evidence synthesis,** and **Pragmatic clinical trial.**

Validation : One of 14 terms in the contributor roles taxonomy that gives credit for replication or reproducibility of results. *Also see* **CRediT.**

Validity (internal validity) : The degree to which the effects of trial intervention are likely to approximate the 'truth' for the participants recruited in the sample, i.e., are the trial results free of bias? It is a prerequisite for applicability (external validity) of a trial's findings. It is distinct from research integrity flaws that arise from research misconduct and questionable research practices. *Also see* **Bias, Quality of a study, Effect,** and **External validity.**

Version of record : The final published version of a manuscript (following peer review, editorial assessments and author revisions) in its definitive form with copyediting and typesetting completed, metadata applied, and DOI (digital object identifier) allocated. It may appear as an online accepted manuscript prior to the release of the version of record. Depending on the copyright agreement, the version of record may be immediately open access, or there may be an embargo period. *Also see* **Open science, Open access, Preprint,** and **Peer review.**

Visualization : One of 14 terms in the contributor roles taxonomy that gives credit for the preparation of data presentation. *Also see* **CRediT.**

WAME : World Association of Medical Editors. Among other things, it aims to improve editorial standards and promote professionalism in medical editing through education, self-criticism and self-regulation (wame.org). *Also see* **Journal, ICMJE,** and **COPE.**

Whistleblower : An individual, also known as the complainant, who reports a possible current or past breach of research integrity, making an allegation of research misconduct or questionable research practice. Complaints ought to be made in good faith with reasonable belief or evidence of wrongdoing. The complaint made may be found or there may be no case to answer on investigation. *Also see* **Data sleuthing, GCP, Questionable research practice, Research integrity,** and **Research misconduct.**

Withdrawals : Participants who do not fully comply with the intervention, cross over and receive an alternative intervention, choose to drop out, or are lost to follow-up. An adverse event may be the reason for withdrawal. *Also see* **Adverse event, Attrition bias, Intention-to-treat analysis,** and **Sensitivity analysis.**

Writing original draft : One of 14 terms in the contributor roles taxonomy that gives credit for the preparation of the initial draft of the manuscript to be submitted for publication. *Also see* **CRediT.**

Index

A

ACTIVE, *see* Authors and Consumers Together Impacting on eVidencE
Adverse event, 81–83, 85, 121
AI, *see* Artificial intelligence
Allocation sequence, 11, 12, 98
AllTrials, 24, 70, 98
Anonymization, 33, 105
Applicability, 11, 14, 53
Applied research, 17, 50
Artificial intelligence (AI), 96, 97, 136
Attrition bias, 13, 101
Audit, 30, 56, 79
Authors and Consumers Together Impacting on eVidencE (ACTIVE), 63, 122
Authorship, 32–33; *see also* Contributorship
  abuse, 32, 117, 158
  academic implications, 113
  acknowledgments, 121–122
  citizens as co-authors, 122–123
  coercion authorship, 118
  collaboration authorship, 18
  corresponding author, 113
  criteria, 114
  defined, 112
  features, trial collaborations, 112–113
  ghost, 118
  gift, 118
  healthcare research landscape, 113
  issues and considerations, 121
  last author, 113
  multicenter trials, 119–121
  orphan, 118
  unethical, 117–118

B

Balance of probabilities, 151
Basic laboratory research, 17, 50
Biomedical journals, 17
Biomedical research, 2

C

Case report form, 81
ChatGPT, 122
Cherry-picking, 35, 72
Chief investigator, 79, 120
Citizen science, 40, 62, 64, 84, 122
Clinical
  equipoise, 49
  investigator, 36, 55, 81, 119

practice guideline, 128, 129
research ecosystem, 36–38
The Coalition for Advancing Research Assessment (CoARA), 32–33
CoARA, *see* The Coalition for Advancing Research Assessment
Coercion authorship, 118
Coercive citation practices, 97
Collaboration authorship, 118
Committee on Publication Ethics (COPE), 28, 94, 117, 143
Complaints, 144–148
Composite outcomes, 21, 67
Confidentiality, 146
Confirmatory trial, 3, 14
Conflict of interests, 59, 68, 89, 109, 123, 141, 147
Consent exemption, 55
Consort, 103, 155
Contributor roles taxonomy (CRediT), 75, 112, 115, 116
Contributorship, 115; *see also* Authorship
Coordinated campaigns, 24, 70
COPE, *see* Committee on Publication Ethics
Core outcomes set, 64
Corresponding author, 113
Corrigendum, 1, 19, 140, 153
CRediT, *see* Contributor roles taxonomy
Critical appraisal, 17–18, 23

D

Data
  deidentification, 33
  sharing, 105–106
  sleuthing, 98, 131, 143
Database development, 81
Data monitoring committee (DMC), 85–87, 121
The Declaration on Research Assessment (DORA), 33
DELTA, *see* Difference ELicitation in TriAls
Difference ELicitation in TriAls (DELTA), 69, 103
Digital Object Identifier (DOI), 95, 115
Directory of Open Access Journals (DOAJ), 95
Discrimination, 150
Disease burden studies, 47
Disease-related risks, 52
DMC, *see* Data Monitoring Committee
DOAJ, *see* Directory of Open Access Journals
DOI, *see* Digital Object Identifier
DORA, *see* The Declaration on Research Assessment

Double-blinding peer review, 107
Drug regulatory approval, 4–5

E
Effectiveness vs. efficacy, 14–16, 22, 48
EMA, see European Medicines Agency
Epidemiological methods, 47
Equality, 150
    diversity, 54
Enhancing the QUAlity and Transparency Of health
        Research (EQUATOR), 66, 103, 155
EQUATOR, see Enhancing the QUAlity and
        Transparency Of health Research
Equipoise, 49, 67
Ethical justification, see Scientific, justification
Ethics, 27, 43; see also Human research ethics
    dumping, 117
European Medicines Agency (EMA), 15, 82
Evidence-based medicine, 1, 9, 126, 129, 155, 156
Evidence strength, 130
Evidence synthesis
    defined, 6, 19, 21, 47, 126, 128
    nomenclature, 128
    open science, 140
    randomized clinical trials, 126, 130
    systematic review, 129
    trial integrity, 131–132
    trial integrity assessment, 134–137
    trials, 19–23, 126, 127
    usefulness, 137–140
Explanatory trial, 3, 14, 50
Expression of concern, 5, 38, 44, 131, 150
External validity, 11, 53

F
FAIR, see Findable, Accessible, Interoperable and
        Reusable
Fake peer review, 96
False allegations, 102
FDA, see Food and Drug Administration
Financial conflicts of interests, 102
Findable, Accessible, Interoperable and Reusable
        (FAIR), 106
Fitness-to-practice investigation, 156–157
Food and Drug Administration (FDA), 15
Forest plot, 19, 130, 133
Formal complaint, 146
Formal peer review, 97, 143
Formal research misconduct investigation, 148–152
Freedom of information, 153
Funders, 6, 17, 38–39, 56, 95
Funnel plot, 130, 134

G
GCP, see Good Clinical Practice
Generative Artificial Intelligence (AI), 114, 122
Generative Pretrained Transformer (ChatGPT), 122
Genuine vs. predatory publishing, 96
Ghost authorship, 118
Gift authorship, 118
Gold open access, 95
Good Clinical Practice (GCP), 27, 28, 56, 79,
        143, 144
Good Publication Practice (GPP), 122
GPP, see Good Publication Practice
Green open access, 95
GRIPP, see Guidance for Reporting Involvement of
        Patients and the Public
Group allocation, 12
Guest authorship, 118
Guidance for Reporting Involvement of Patients
        and the Public (GRIPP), 60, 122

H
Healthcare professionals, 58
Healthcare research, 2
    integrity, 38–39
Heterogeneity, 129, 133, 136
h(Hirsh)-index, 32
Highly prolific authorship, 118
Human research ethics
    autonomy, 43, 44
    beneficence, 43, 45
    blatant exploitation, 44
    committees, 45–46
        members, 53
        privacy protection, 53
        risk to participants, 51–53
    justice, 43, 45
    non-maleficence, 43, 45

I
ICMJE, see International Committee of Medical
        Journal Editors
Impact factor, 33
Inadequate citation practices, 109
Independent data monitoring committee, 85
Independent oversight, 82–83
Individual participant data (IPD) meta-
        analysis, 53, 106, 126, 128, 136
Informed consent, 54, 56–58
Inspection, 56, 79
Institution, 6, 28, 38, 45, 71, 78, 113, 137, 143
Institutional review board (IRB), 43; see also
        Human research ethics

Instrument, 135
Integrity, 136
  appraisal, 100
  assessment, 130, 137
  flaws, 142–144
Intellectual honesty, 29, 33–34
Intention-to-treat, 12, 72, 73
Internal validity, 11, 18, 36, 48
International Committee of Medical Journal Editors
    (ICMJE), 32, 70, 71, 88, 94, 112, 114
Intervention-related risks, 52
Intervention's effect, 50
Invented authorship, 118
IPD meta-analysis, see Individual participant data
    meta-analysis
Irresponsible research conduct, 145

J
Journals, 6, 17, 28, 39, 70, 84, 92, 112, 137, 142
  authors' instructions, 103–104
  openness, 107–108

L
Last author, 113
Local research ethics committees, 46

M
Mapping review, 128
Measurement bias, 13
Meta-analysis, 19–20, 84, 128, 129
  IPD, 126, 128, 136
  network, 128
  retracted and republished, 132
Meta-regression, 130, 136
Misconduct, 29, 137, 142
Misconduct investigation
  correction to research record, 154–156
  defamation claim, 147
  filing and assessing complaint, 144–148
  formal research, 148–152
  integrity flaws, 142–144
  respondent trialists, 152–153
  sanctions, 153–154
Multi-arm multistage trial, 138
Multi-country trials, 46

N
National research integrity policies, 154
Network meta-analysis, 128
Non-maleficence, 83
Non-randomized trials, 51
Nuremberg Code, 44

O
OASPA, see Open Access Scholarly Publishers
    Association
Open Access Scholarly Publishers Association
    (OASPA), 95
Open peer review, 107
Open science, 2, 39–40, 53, 62, 92, 140
ORCID, see Unique author identifier
Orphan authorship, 118
Outcome adjudication committee, 82

P
Paid authorship, 118
Paper mills, 94–97, 117
Participants, 51, 63
Paternalistic medicine, 62, 122
Patient communities, 62
Peer-reviewed journal, 17
Performance bias, 13
Per-protocol analysis, 16
p-hacking, 92
Pilot trial, 3, 50, 64
Plagiarism, 99
Policy, 8, 37, 146
Post-publication scientific record, 96
Power, statistical, 58, 117, 146
Pragmatic trial, 4
Pragmatism, 16–17, 138, 139
Precision of effect, 11, 48
Predatory journals, 95
Predatory publishing, 95
Preprint, 75, 95
Pre-review, 143
Pre-specified statistical analysis plan, 74
Principle, 7, 27, 44
Procedure, 8, 37, 146
Professional regulatory body, 154
Proof-of-concept study, 3
Prospective registration, 70–71
Pseudonymization, 33; see also Anonymization
Pseudo-randomized trials, 133
Publication bias, 34, 129
Publication process manipulation, 107
Public documentation, 62, 87–88
Publicly accessible registration, 71
Publishing, 94–97
Publish-or-perish academic culture, 32–33, 113
PubMed, 5, 17–18, 37, 93

Q
Quasi-randomized studies, 133
Questionable research practices, 29, 137, 142, 145

R
Random error, 11
Randomization, 12
    subversion of, 35–36
Randomized clinical trial, 3
    arm, 9
    biases, 13
    components, 10
    confirmatory trial, 3
    drug regulatory approval, 4–5
    education and training, 7
    effect estimation, 16
    explanatory trial, 3
    intervention effectiveness, 11
    interventions, 15–16
    outcomes, 16
    participants, 15
    pilot trial, 3
    pragmatic trial, 4
Recklessness, 29
Regulator, 6, 7, 15, 59, 72, 82, 105
Reporting checklists, 103
Research
    conduct, 29–32
    culture, 40–41, 159
    gap, 22, 46, 63, 75, 100, 140
    governance, 28, 46, 78, 79, 143
    integrity, 6, 7, 23, 27, 99, 131, 142, 144
    integrity failure, 29–32
    misconduct investigation, 144, 145
    need, 22, 46, 63, 75, 100
    priority, 21, 46, 63, 75, 100, 140
Respondent, 146
    trialists, 152–153
Responsible contribution, 42
Responsible research conduct, 27–28
Restoration, 24–25
Restoring Invisible and Abandoned Trials (RIAT), 24, 70, 98
Retracted papers, 97
Retractions, 1, 5–6, 33, 44, 131, 147, 155–157

S
SAGER, see Sex and Gender Equity in Research
Sanctions, 153–154
Scientific
    justification, 47–51
    uncertainty, 34–35
    virtue, 29
Scientific, Technical, and Medical (STM), 17, 37, 94
Scoping reviews, 128
Selection bias, 13, 36

Selective outcome reporting, 34, 70, 132
Self-regulating community, 94–97
Sensitivity analysis, 72, 132
Sex and Gender Equity in Research (SAGER), 103
Shared decision-making, 55
Site principal investigator, 55, 81, 119
Societies, 36, 158
Space science, 105
SPIRIT, see Standard Protocol Items Recommended for Interventional Trials
Sponsor, 59
Stakeholder engagement, 47
Stakeholder organizations, 6–7
Standard, 7, 27, 44
Standard Protocol Items Recommended for Interventional Trials (SPIRIT), 66, 103
Statistical analysis plan, 71–74
Statistical power, 12, 67, 106
Study quality assessment, 130
Subgroup analysis, 130, 135
Surrogate outcomes, 16
Suspension, 152
Systematic review, 19, 84, 126, 128, 129
    trial integrity assessment, 132–135

T
Target condition, 15, 49, 64
Template for Intervention Description and Replication (TIDieR), 103
Theoretical efficacy, 14
TIDieR, see Template for Intervention Description and Replication
Timely open publication, 41
TOP, see Transparency and Openness Promotion
Trail effects, 129
Transparency and Openness Promotion (TOP), 25, 91, 103, 104
Transparency in research, 23, 40, 62, 90, 108, 133, 157
Treatment network, 130, 138
Trial integrity, 131–132
Trial integrity assessment
    controversial aspects, 137
    developments for, 135–136
    steps of, 134
    systematic review, 132–135
Trialist, 6, 7, 46, 78, 146
Trial management group, 78–81, 120, 121
Trial priority, 46–47
Trial protocol, 64–68
Trial sample size estimation, 68–69

Trial's lifecycle, 126, 127
Trial statistical analysis, 73–74
Trial Steering Committee (TSC), 83–85, 121
TSC, *see* Trial Steering Committee

U
Umbrella review, 128, 138
Unethical authorship, 117–118
Unique author identifier (ORCID), 115
Untrustworthy COVID-19 trials, 93
Untrustworthy trials, 92–93

Usefulness of evidence syntheses, 137–140
Usefulness of trials, 21–23, 48, 64, 100, 119

V
Variance, 135
Version of record, 95, 154

W
WAME, *see* World Association of Medical Editors
Whistleblower, 141, 142, 144, 146, 147
World Association of Medical Editors (WAME), 37, 94

Printed in the United States
by Baker & Taylor Publisher Services